Perioperative Care, Anaesthesia, Pain Management and Intensive Care

AN ILLUSTRATED COLOUR TEXT

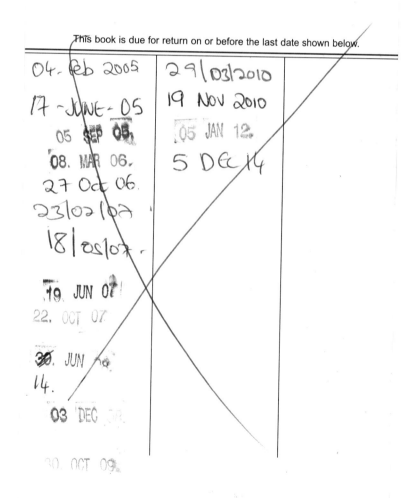
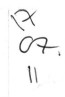

Commissioning Editor: Michael Parkinson
Project Development Manager: Lynn Watt
Project Controller: Nancy Arnott
Designer: Sarah Russell

Perioperative Care, Anaesthesia, Pain Management and Intensive Care

AN ILLUSTRATED COLOUR TEXT

Michael Avidan MBBCh FCA
Assistant Professor
Anaesthesiology and Intensive Care
Washington University School of Medicine
St Louis, Missouri,
USA

Andrea M.R. Harvey MB ChB MSc FRCA
Consultant in Anaesthetics and Pain Management
Department of Anaesthetics,
Aberdeen Royal Infirmary,
Foresterhill, Aberdeen
UK

Illustrated by Graeme Chambers

José Ponte DIC, PhD, FRCA
Senior Lecturer in Anaesthetics and Honorary
Consultant for King's Healthcare
Guy's, Kings and St Thomas's School of Medicine
London
UK

Julia Wendon MBChB, FRCP
Senior Lecturer and Honorary Consultant
Institute of Liver Studies
King's College Hospital
London
UK

Robert Ginsburg BSc, MB, BS, FRCA
Anaesthetic Consultant
King's College Hospital
London
and
Associate Dean of Postgraduate Medicine
London Department of Postgraduate Medical and
Dental Education
London
UK

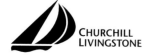
CHURCHILL
LIVINGSTONE

EDINBURGH   LONDON   NEW YORK   PHILADELPHIA   ST LOUIS   SYDNEY   TORONTO   2003

CHURCHILL LIVINGSTONE
An imprint of Elsevier Science Limited

First published 2003

ISBN 0443 06410 5

British Library Cataloguing in Publication Data
A catalogue record for this book is available from the British Library

Library of Congress Cataloging in Publication Data
A catalog record for this book is available from the Library of Congress

> **Note**
> Medical knowledge is constantly changing. As new information
> becomes available, changes in treatment, procedures, equipment
> and the use of drugs become necessary. The authors and the
> publishers have, as far as it is possible, taken care to ensure that
> the information given in this text is accurate and up to date.
> However, readers are strongly advised to confirm that the
> information, especially with regard to drug usage, complies with
> the latest legislation and standards of practice.

 your source for books,
journals and multimedia
in the health sciences

www.elsevierhealth.com

The
publisher's
policy is to use
**paper manufactured
from sustainable forests**

Printed in China by RDC Group Limited

Preface

Surgery has changed dramatically over the past 200 years. Previously morbidity and mortality were high, yet today most people expect not only to survive an operation, but to do so with minimal discomfort and disruption to their lives. As operative interventions become more ambitious, older and sicker people are now undergoing major surgery. This has provided impetus to the burgeoning specialties of Anaesthesia, Pain Management and Intensive Care.

Perioperative care is a challenging and rewarding area of patient management. The Illustrated Colour Textbook is intended for medical students and doctors who wish to improve their approach to perioperative management. In keeping with other books in this series, topics are covered in double-page spreads. There are summary points and clinical case studies to encourage retention of key points and appreciation of concepts. This book is not intended as an exhaustive reference and readers are encouraged to read further. Recent articles from mainstream international journals are suggested in the further reading section to supplement most topics in the book.

We hope that you enjoy reading this Illustrated Colour Text.

Missouri 2002

M.A. A.H.

Acknowledgements

Many people have helped this book's evolution into its final printed form. It is a pleasure to acknowledge the contribution of the publishing staff at Elsevier Science in the production of this book, in particular Lynn Watt and Sarah Keer-Keer who patiently guided our efforts and provided tactful criticism. Without their constant feedback, support and insightful editorial comments, this book would not have been completed. The impact of this book owes much to the illustrations. We are grateful to Graeme Chambers for his clear and creative figures.

We would also like to give special thanks for the contributions made by Dr Nicola Jones (HIV and other viruses, Antibiotic prophylaxis and Postoperative infection), Dr Emma Alcock (Practical Procedures, Brain death and Organ Donation) and Dr Jonathan Berry (Resuscitation sections) and the students from King's College Medical School listed overleaf.

We received valued advice and assistance in the compilation of the varied photographic material that appears throughout the book. Readers will have no difficulty distinguishing between the professional photographs and the efforts of the authors. We are grateful especially to David Langdon (Senior Medical Photographer at King's College Hospital), Molly Hedley, Sue Berry and Lisa Tombling (Resuscitation Training Officers at King's College Hospital) and the Medical Photography Departments at King's College Hospital and the John Radcliffe Hospital (Oxford).

Finally our thanks go to the many staff members and patients at King's College Hospital in London, Barnes Jewish Hospital in St Louis and Aberdeen Royal Infirmary, who kindly agreed to their photographs appearing in the book.

Michael Avidan and Andrea Harvey

Contributors

Apart from the authors listed on the cover of the book, three doctors have made major contributions to the book.

Dr Nicola Jones wrote or edited the sections on HIV and other viruses, Antibiotic prophylaxis and Postoperative infection.

Dr Emma Alcock wrote the sections on Practical procedures and Brain death and organ donation.

Dr Jonathan Berry co-authored the Resuscitation sections.

The following is a list of the students who contributed to this book and the sections that they helped to write, in chapter order.

Judith Cheong-Leen	Perioperative safety
	Preoperative assessment
Rajkumar Rajendram	Cardiac disease
	Hypertension
Juliet Drew	Thrombophilia and bleeding tendency
Sabina Hashmy	Obesity
	Alcohol and substance abuse
Lan-Anh Le	Pulmonary disease
	Pregnancy and childbirth

Tom Healy	Techniques of anaesthesia
Colin Shackell	Acid–base abnormalities
	Fluid management
Richard Johnston	HIV and other viruses
	Postoperative neurological complications
Anuj Bahl	The stress response
	Postoperative cardiovascular complications
Riyaz Patel	Sedation
	Postoperative pulmonary complications
Daniel Crespi	Blood products
	Postoperative bleeding
Rachel Fettiplace	Intraoperative complications
	Perioperative infection
Rebecca Boreham	Local anaesthesia
	Regional analgesia
Trushar Bavalia	Complementary medicine and analgesia
	ABCDs of pain management problems
Raju Ahluwalia	Infants and children
	Pain in the young and the old
Ross Hunter	Reasons for ICU admission
	Monitoring of the ICU patient
Susannah Woodrow	Resuscitation

Contents

Clinical case comments

Further reading

Index and abbreviations

The history of modern perioperative care

Many chapters on the historical development of a subject, included within a textbook for the sake of completeness, describe the evolution of that subject in a linear way, starting with earliest events and then moving in sequence to the present day. However, history rarely works that way. More often, it is a combination of coincidence, observation, curiosity and need, spiced with flashes of the inspiration and insight that provide the real impetus to progress.

Occasionally, a technique or device is introduced in advance of its time, its true merit being appreciated decades or generations later. Often, it is the development of one technique that facilitates enormous strides in another unrelated field. Local anaesthetics would not have achieved their importance without the development of the syringe and hypodermic needle. Similarly, it is unlikely that the laryngeal mask airway would have achieved the success it has without the introduction of the hypnotic agent propofol.

Few major advances in surgery would have been possible without contemporaneous breakthroughs in anaesthesia, intensive care, analgesia, fluid management, pharmacology,

understanding of physiology, antiseptic techniques and technology.

In Fig. 1, there is an attempt to depict graphically some of the inter-related developments that have occurred alongside the huge strides that have been made in surgery over the past few hundred years. The detail is by no means exhaustive. Nonetheless, illustrated are some of the milestones which have facilitated the march from crude surgical interventions to the modern-day array of surgical techniques, including day surgery, minimally invasive surgery, major organ transplantation and microsurgery. Over the past 50 years, anaesthesia, critical care and pain management have all emerged as specialities in their own right.

Anaesthetic techniques

The first display by Morton of general anaesthesia, using ether at the Massachusetts General Hospital, signified a major advance. Surgery on awake subjects had been associated with

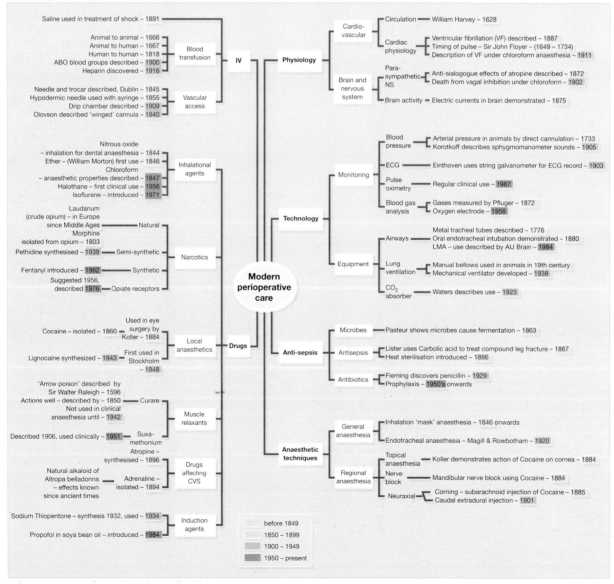

Fig. 1 **Spider diagram map depicting some of the multifaceted advances in perioperative care.**

terrible suffering and high mortality. General anaesthesia provided the opportunity to carry out life-saving surgical interventions which had been previously impossible. Nonetheless, drugs like ether and chloroform were associated with high morbidity and convalescence was long following early surgery and anaesthesia.

The advent of regional anaesthetic techniques with local anaesthetic agents provided alternatives and adjuncts to general anaesthesia. Combining general and regional anaesthesia has recently been suggested to result in improved outcome and patient comfort.

Over the last century, anaesthesia has become extremely safe and even the sickest patients may be offered surgery with the expectation of a favourable outcome.

Pharmacology

The development of safer and non-inflammable inhalational agents such as halothane allowed massive strides to be made in surgery. Over the last 50 years, the concept of balanced anaesthesia, incorporating a range of analgesic drugs, muscle relaxants and hypnotic agents, has further sophisticated perioperative care.

Exciting molecular biology and genetic research by the likes of Franks and Lieb has advanced our understanding of the mechanisms of anaesthesia. In the future the possibility exists of administering anaesthetic drugs which act at specific receptors and which are tailored to individuals according to their genotypes.

Intravenous fluids

The simple administration of sterile intravenous crystalloids, such as normal saline and Hartman's, has allowed an extended the surgical repertoire. Blood volume and fluid losses may be replaced during surgery and in the postoperative period when patients are unable to drink. Without the safe transfusion of blood and blood products, many major surgical procedures could not be undertaken.

The future promises oxygen-carrying alternatives to human blood, which would eliminate many of the hazards of blood-product transfusion, such as anaphylaxis and viral infection.

Physiology

Without an advanced understanding of human physiology, it would be impossible to provide life support during anaesthesia and for patients in intensive care units. Anaesthetists and intensivists are particularly aware of the functioning of vital organ systems and interventions are frequently warranted to maintain adequate cardiac output, to support gas exchange in the lungs and to prevent the failure of organs such as the liver and kidneys.

The central nervous system is the target of anaesthetic and analgesic strategies. We constantly strive to refine our interventions so that disturbances to essential physiological functions are minimized.

Technology

A myriad of technological advances allow physicians to interpret precisely physiological parameters and apply specific therapeutic interventions.

Cardiac output may be gauged through surrogate measures, such as automatic blood-pressure devices and capnography, while the pulmonary artery catheter allows direct measurement. Recent research suggests that the combination of the capnograph and the pulse oximeter detect more than 90% of critical incidents occurring during anaesthesia.

The ability to provide an artificial airway, coupled with assisted ventilation of the lungs, has allowed the use of neuromuscular blocking drugs ('muscle relaxants') and has been one of the most important developments in advanced life-support.

Non-invasive monitoring of heart function and cardiac output is already available, and reliable monitors of brain function, which would constitute a major advance in general anaesthesia, are in the offing.

Antibiotics and antisepsis

The 'germ' theory of disease has revolutionized the practice of medicine and dispelled numerous myths. Antiseptic techniques and antimicrobial drugs, such as penicillin, have incalculably improved surgical outcome. In the pre-antibiotic era, the risk of dying from an infectious complication of surgery was substantial. The mortality rate following amputation decreased from 46% in 1867 to 15% with the introduction of aseptic techniques. Prophylactic antibiotic usage from the 1950s onwards has significantly decreased postoperative infectious morbidity. However, this is one area where, despite major advances, the ominous emergence of multi-drug-resistant organisms may strike a crippling blow against the care of the surgical patient.

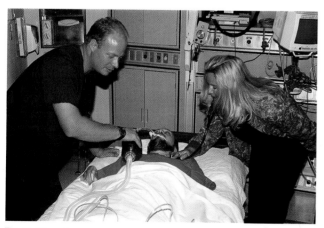

Fig. 2 **There is an apocryphal story about Scandinavian medical students taking turns to provide assisted ventilation to polio sufferers during an epidemic in Denmark in the 1950s.** This epidemic provided a major impetus to the development of mechanical ventilators.

> ### History of perioperative care
> - There have been major strides in surgery over the past 200 years.
> - These advances have been facilitated by developments in related disciplines.
> - Anaesthesia, critical care and pain management have emerged as independent specialities.
> - Current and future advances will ensure that patients may undergo major surgery with increasing safety and comfort.

Perioperative safety

Apprehension about surgery and anaesthesia is a common and natural response. Risk is present in most human experiences. Surgery and anaesthesia are not exceptions.

It is important to identify specific risk-factors and to reassure patients that every effort will be made to minimize risks and maximize their safety. General anaesthesia is a vulnerable state during which complete trust is placed in the anaesthetist. Patients, whether under general anaesthesia or heavy sedation, are incapable of protecting themselves and they rely on the anaesthetist to act as their advocate. In assessing the risk to each individual patient, it is necessary to consider the patient's health and quality of life and to question whether the proposed benefits of surgery outweigh the attendant risks.

Mortality attributable to anaesthesia itself is rare, with studies suggesting that the incidence is between 1 in 100 000 and 1 in 300 000. While major complications are rare, minor complications occur more frequently and are often not considered by the patient (see Table 1 and Fig. 1).

Table 1 **Perioperative risks for the patient**	
Major risks (unlikely)	**Minor risks (more likely)**
Death	Pain
Neurological injury	Minor infection
Nerve damage	Minor allergy
Eye damage	Blood transfusion reaction
Awareness	Adverse drug reaction
Thrombosis	Nausea
Anaphylaxis	Tooth damage
Infection	

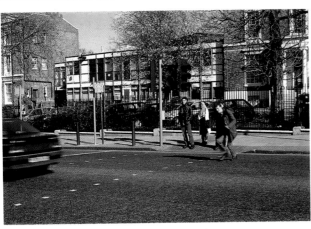

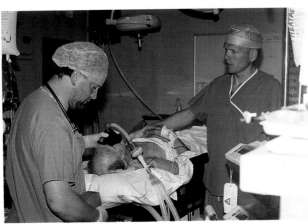

Fig. 1 **Who is at greater risk?**

Consent

Part of obtaining informed consent for a procedure involves providing patients with an honest appraisal about the risks, so that they are in a position to decide whether they wish to undergo the proposed surgical intervention (Fig. 2). Patients should receive any information to which a reasonable person in their position would be likely to attach significance. Similarly, where options exist these should be presented fully, thereby empowering patients to make crucial decisions.

Discussions about risks and patients' decisions should be well documented in the notes. Patients who have given consent can still claim compensation if they suffer an injury during a procedure that has not been explained to them as a potential risk.

Frequently asked questions about consent

What information should be given?
Sufficient information should be provided to enable the patient to make an informed decision. Areas to cover include diagnosis, prognosis, options for management, name of doctor in charge, likelihood that the procedure will be a success, possibility of side effects or adverse outcome, possibility of additional problems coming to light during surgery and how those would be dealt with.

Should information ever be withheld?
Information that may assist a decision must not be withheld from the patient even at the request of relatives or friends.

How much time should be allowed?
Allow the patient sufficient time to reflect on the diagnosis and proposed management. Allow time for questions.

Who obtains consent?
The doctor providing the treatment has the responsibility for obtaining consent. This task can be delegated to a suitably trained and qualified colleague, who has sufficient knowledge of the diagnosis and treatment plan.

What happens in emergencies?
Where consent cannot be obtained, medical treatment can be provided to save life or prevent deterioration in a patient's

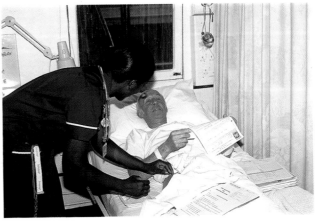

Fig. 2 **A patient giving informed consent for a procedure.**

condition. The treatment given should be explained to the patient as soon as possible.

Oral or written?

Consent should be written if possible.

Decreasing the risks

Preoperative

A thorough preoperative assessment is required, including history, examination and risk-assessment. This is considered in more detail on page 6.

Perioperative

It is essential that the patient's identity is confirmed. On admission patients are given identity bracelets with their name, hospital number and date of birth. More than one bracelet is usually applied to allow removal during venous or arterial cannulation. The anaesthetist must ensure that the correct patient is anaesthetized and that the details on the theatre list correspond with those on the identity bracelet and in the clinical notes. It is the responsibility of the operating team to mark the operative site. It should be checked that consent has been obtained for the particular procedure to be performed.

Confirmation that patients have not eaten and have received prescribed medications is important before embarking upon anaesthesia. The anaesthetic equipment must be checked and should meet the standards laid out by the Association of Anaesthetists of Great Britain and Ireland. An emergency supply of oxygen and a simple means to provide ventilation should always be available.

Alarm limits of monitors should be set to appropriate levels and ought not to be disabled at any time during the procedure. The choice of monitoring is informed by the patient's specific risk, as well as the extent of surgery. There is a minimum standard of monitoring for all patients undergoing anaesthesia, which includes pulse oximetry, inspired oxygen analysis, blood pressure measurement, electrocardiography and capnography.

When drugs are administered, the drug name, dosage, patients name band and expiry date should be checked. The anaesthetist must stay alert to various unpredictable hazards such as hypoxia, hypercarbia, hypotension, blood loss, hypothermia and awareness (see Table 2). In order to fulfil this role adequately the anaesthetist must be present throughout the whole operation.

Postoperative

The transfer of a patient from the operating theatre to the recovery area should be supervised to prevent trauma, hypoxia or accidental disconnection of drains or catheters. Anaesthetists should not leave patients until they are awake and capable of protecting their own airways. Patients should be haemodynamically stable and pain and nausea should be well controlled.

A formal handover to the recovery staff is mandatory, complete with written and verbal instructions for postoperative care, accompanied by the anaesthetic record and details of the surgery.

Health worker safety

Doctors and other medical staff are not exempt from risk. They must take precautions to protect themselves from physical injury and litigation. All health workers should take the following precautions.

- Effective communication in many cases can save misunderstandings and avoid patient complaints.
- Comprehensive notes should be taken at the preoperative assessment and during anaesthesia. Surgeons should detail all procedures which have been performed. All notes must be legible.
- All staff should undergo regular training and ensure that they are qualified to do the job required of them.
- Doctors should only perform procedures within their capabilities.
- Advice from colleagues and senior staff should be sought when necessary.
- All doctors should have medicolegal insurance.
- When performing an invasive procedure, universal precautions must be taken. These include wearing gloves and treating all body fluids as a potential hazard.

Clinical case 1

A patient awaiting minor surgery approaches his GP with concerns. His grandfather died during surgery and his friend had a tooth broken during an operation last year. In addition, he has read a newspaper article telling the story of someone 'waking on the table'. He also has a penicillin allergy and fears that while he is asleep someone may administer it.

See comment on page 122.

Table 2 **The role of the anaesthetist**

	Perceived	Actual
Who is the anaesthetist	Non-medically-trained technician	Specialist doctor with a minimum of 6 years postgraduate training
What is the anaesthetist's role?	Injects hypnotic drugs and then relaxes	Analogous to an airline pilot – not always intervening but constantly vigilant in case of an emergency
What other roles does the anaesthetist have?	None	Pain-relief, preoperative assessment and optimization, intensive care management, resuscitation, labour analgesia, teaching and research
What occurs during anaesthesia?	People often experience pain, awareness and nightmares	Anaesthesia is usually safe and uneventful

---

Perioperative safety

- All surgery and anaesthesia is associated with some risk.
- Risks are specific to each individual patient.
- Patients require an honest appraisal of the risks.
- Informed consent is required from all patients (except in extreme circumstances).
- Anaesthesia is a vulnerable state during which patients trust the anaesthetist entirely.
- Everything possible must be done to ensure the safety of the patient.
- Health workers should take precautions to protect themselves.

Preoperative assessment

Rapport

A preoperative assessment should be a two-way exchange of information, with patients feeling comfortable to ask questions. Providing a good understanding of proposed surgery allays many patients' concerns. Positive rapport with staff promotes confidence and reduces anxiety (see Fig. 1).

Many patients simply require information and reassurance, rather than sedative premedication. Written informed consent should be obtained. This is dealt with in chapter 4.

History

A full history should be taken paying particular attention to the following:

Previous surgery and anaesthesia This may highlight areas of potential difficulty, including adverse reactions to particular drugs, difficulties with tracheal intubation and postoperative pain or nausea. Such information informs anaesthetic technique and prevents repeats of previous complications.

Medication A list of medications allows physicians to anticipate drug interactions and provides insight into medical problems.

Allergies It is important to distinguish between what the patient may describe as an allergy, but what is actually a known side-effect of a medication.

Dentition

Dental damage may occur, usually during direct laryngoscopy. Patients should be told of the potential risks ranging from chipping to possible fractures, the upper incisors being most vulnerable. Loose teeth, caps, crowns and dentures should be noted and if the teeth are in poor condition a dental opinion may be sought prior to surgery.

Upper respiratory tract infections (URTIs)

During everyday life the common cold is little more than a nuisance. Under general anaesthesia, however, there is increased risk of life-threatening bronchospasm and laryngospasm following instrumentation of the larynx or pharynx. Postoperative coughing may place strain on sutures. It is therefore considered sensible to delay elective surgery until patients have recovered from the acute phase of URTIs. This is particularly true for children and the elderly.

Systems review

Special attention should be given to the cardiovascular and respiratory systems. Many diseases affecting these systems may be worsened during and after surgery. Such conditions include ischaemic heart disease, heart failure, chronic obstructive pulmonary disease and asthma.

Effort tolerance may be one of the most important determinants of a patient's ability to cope with the stress imposed by surgery and anaesthesia. Additionally, other systemic disorders including obesity, diabetes and liver failure have important implications for perioperative care.

Examination

Evidence of heart failure, uncontrolled hypertension, congenital cardiac disease, heart valve pathology and arrythmias should be elicited. Walking with a patient up two flights of stairs may reveal cardiorespiratory compromise.

Diminished respiratory function as evidenced by wheezing, chest crackles, cyanosis and tachypnoea may require further investigation. The peak flowmeter, a simple bedside test, provides valuable information. The upper airway should be examined for anatomical abnormalities that may lead to difficulties with tracheal intubation. These include tracheal deviation, limited mouth opening and decreased neck mobility.

Investigations

A thorough history and examination informs special investigations. It is neither cost-effective nor helpful to routinely order a battery of tests. Such tests are of value only if they provide information that cannot be gleaned clinically and that may influence management. For minor surgery, special investigations escalate costs without altering management. This applies even to patients with serious diseases.

Urine analysis is a cheap bedside investigation and may be useful in suggesting undiagnosed diabetes mellitus, in detecting proteinuria and in alerting to urinary tract infections.

Haemoglobin measurement is indicated before surgery where major blood loss is anticipated. It may be justifiable in the elderly and in menstruating women or when there is reason to suspect anaemia. When there is concern about abnormal clotting, platelet count and coagulation studies should be performed.

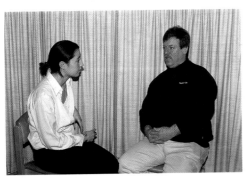
(a)

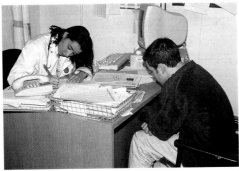
(b)

Fig. 1 **(a) Good communication and rapport. (b) Lack of interest and distance.**

Urea, creatinine and electrolytes could be pursued in the event of dehydration, renal dysfunction or suspected electrolyte abnormalities. Women of childbearing age should have a pregnancy test to prevent teratogen administration.

There is controversy surrounding routine chest X-rays and electrocardiograms. As with other investigations, they should only be requested for specific indications.

The guiding principle for all special investigations is that they should only be ordered if the information may alter management. For example, lung function tests may show whether asthma is optimally controlled. If there is markedly improved lung function following inhaled bronchodilators, elective surgery should be postponed.

Assessing patient fitness

In assessing a patient's suitability for surgery and anaesthesia, it is worth considering the potential benefits of the proposed surgery and deciding whether these outweigh the risks to the patient. It is also important to determine whether medical problems may be improved, in which case it may be prudent to postpone surgery (see Fig. 2).

A classification system (Table 1) describing fitness for surgery was recommended by the American Society of Anesthesiologists (ASA) and is widely used by anaesthetists.

Preoperative management

A treatment plan tailored to the individual should be drawn up. One of the main objectives of premedication is the reduction of anxiety (see Fig. 3). Patients may benefit from an anxiolytic medication, a typical example being a benzodiazepine. Pain-relief is indicated if the patient is in pain before surgery.

Aspiration of gastric contents into the lungs is a potentially fatal complication during surgery. Certain precautions are adopted to minimize this risk. These include fasting for 6–8

Table 1	**Preoperative physical status classification (ASA)**
Class I	Fit and healthy individual
Class II	Patient with mild systemic disease
Class III	Patient with severe systemic disease that is not incapacitating
Class IV	Patient with incapacitating systemic disease which is constantly threatening life
Class V	Moribund patient not expected to survive more than 24 h with or without surgery

hours before anaesthesia and having unrestricted clear fluid intake up to 2 hours before the scheduled operation. For patients without gastrointestinal disorders, a fast for 4 hours represents a negligible risk. Non-particulate antacids, histamine receptor blockers and proton pump inhibitors may be given prior to induction of anaesthesia. Metoclopramide and erythromycin encourage gastric emptying. Despite precautions, certain patients remain at risk for aspiration. Trauma, obesity, gastrointestinal pathology, pregnancy, autonomic dysfunction and opioid medications are associated with impaired gastric emptying.

Clinical case 2

A patient with a history of peptic ulcer disease approaches his doctor before surgery. He is concerned that he may have an increased risk during anaesthesia, and worries about being 'nil by mouth' beforehand.
See comments on page 122.

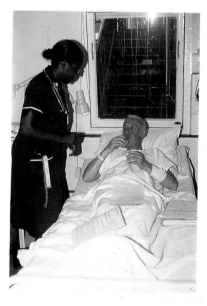

Fig. 3 **Patient receiving temazepam 20 mg before being taken to the operating theatre.**

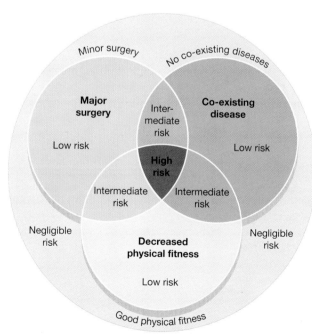

Fig. 2 **Venn diagram for preoperative assessment.**
Three key questions:
1 Is the surgery necessary or is there a less invasive or minor alternative?
2 Can co-existing diseases be treated or improved prior to surgery?
3 Can physical fitness be improved prior to surgery?

Preoperative assessment

- Communication, information and reassurance are more important than anxiolytic drugs.
- History and examination are more useful and cost-effective than special investigations in providing information before surgery.
- Patients are at highest risk of cardiac and respiratory complications. Assessment should focus on these systems.
- Special investigations are indicated only if they may alter management.
- All information gleaned should be clearly documented in the patient's notes.

Perioperative medications

Introduction

Patients presenting for surgery frequently take medications. Doctors should advise which treatments may be continued and which stopped. This decision is sometimes complicated and there may be risks associated both with the cessation and continuation of certain therapies.

The doctor and the patient should make decisions about therapy jointly. Taking some tablets with water before an operation does not increase the risk of aspiration. Generally, people take medications for good reasons, which remain valid around the time of surgery (see Fig. 1). Nonetheless, it is worth considering that the greater the number of administered drugs, the higher the likelihood of an adverse drug reaction.

There are several factors in the perioperative period that may worsen co-existing diseases or precipitate life-threatening crises. Sedative drugs and the anaesthetic state themselves tend to relieve anxiety, lower blood pressure, decrease cardiac

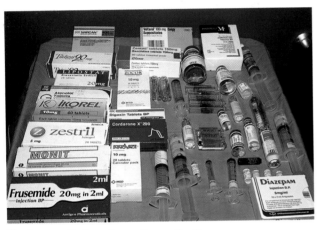

Fig. 1 **Some likely perioperative medications.**

work, and lessen the risk of epileptic seizures. However, the stresses and pain of surgery coupled with possible postoperative complications tend to counteract these salutatory effects. Myocardial ischaemia, hyperglycaemia, ventilatory embarrassment, venous thromboses, seizures, bronchospasm and cognitive dysfunction may occur. There are also important drug interactions which impact upon decisions surrounding therapy (Fig. 2).

Cardiovascular drugs

Ischaemic heart disease is common and the risk of myocardial infarction may be highest up to 3 days following surgery. Most cardiac medications should be continued throughout. β-blockers administered de novo for a week in the perioperative period are associated with decreased mortality for up to 2 years following surgery. ACE inhibitors may be omitted on the morning of surgery as they are associated with intra-operative hypotension.

Aspirin protects against myocardial infarction, thrombotic stroke and postoperative venous thrombosis. However, there may be an increased bleeding risk in those taking aspirin. A realistic compromise is to continue aspirin except when bleeding might have devastating consequences, like eye surgery, neurosurgery, spinal surgery, and possibly cardiac surgery.

Respiratory drugs

Asthma is potentially life threatening. Poorly controlled asthmatics should not have elective surgery. Regular medication should be given before surgery. Nebulized beta-agonist and intravenous steroids may be prescribed as part of

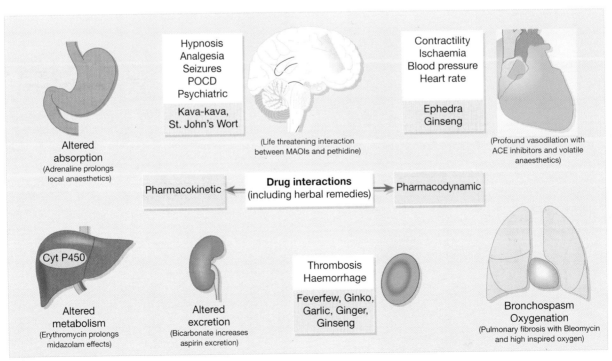

Fig. 2 **Possible drug interactions to be aware of.**

the premedication and adequate sedation and analgesia may be protective. Non-steroidal inflammatory drugs, are best avoided.

Neurological and psychiatric drugs

Epilepsy poses a number of challenges. The seizure threshold is lowered by hypoxia, hypercarbia, sodium derangement, acid–base abnormalities, all of which may occur following surgery. Elevated levels of drugs used to treat epilepsy may themselves cause fits. Phenytoin, carbamazepine and phenobarbitone are all hepatic microsomal enzyme inducers. Anaesthetic drugs may be metabolized more rapidly than anticipated and anaesthetic and analgesic requirements are unpredictable. Safe principles include checking therapeutic drug levels, consulting a neurologist where there is doubt, continuing treatment throughout, avoiding the above physiological derangements, and using sedative and hypnotic drugs with anti-seizure activity like benzodiazepines.

Antidepressants are used to treat chronic pain as well as depression. Selective serotonin reuptake inhibitors are among the most commonly prescribed drugs. Interaction with serotonergic drugs, like pethidine and tramadol, may theoretically precipitate a serotonin syndrome. Monoamine oxidase inhibitors (MAOIs) and tricyclic antidepressants (TCAs) interfere respectively with the metabolism and reuptake of catecholamines. They may cause severe hypertension and arrhythmias, especially if sympathetic stimulants are administered. MAOIs should be withheld for 2 weeks preceding anaesthesia. Pethidine is contraindicated in those taking MAOIs. Neuroleptic drugs, like haloperidol and phenothiazines, are occasionally associated with neurolept malignant syndrome. This resembles malignant hyperthermia clinically. Lithium levels should be checked to avoid toxicity and lithium may be omitted for 24 hours before surgery.

Diabetic medications

The management of diabetes is especially difficult. Patients are fasted and may develop hypoglycaemia. In the postoperative period, the stress response predisposes to hyperglycaemia and ketoacidosis. Metformin carries a theoretical risk of lactic acidosis and should be stopped 48 hours before surgery. An insulin sliding scale may be used instead of oral agents before major surgery. Intravenous dextrose solution on the morning of surgery is advisable to prevent hypoglycaemia. Placing diabetic patients first on operating lists minimizes starvation time and allows for optimal postoperative glycaemic control during daylight hours. Blood glucose and arterial blood gases should be monitored.

Drugs and coagulation

The common indications for anticoagulants include prevention of arterial, venous and atrial thromboses, and prophylaxis against clotting of medical prosthetic devices, like mechanical heart valves. The consequences of clots may be devastating and the perioperative period is associated with an increased thrombotic risk. Where surgery does not carry a high risk of bleeding, anticoagulation should be continued. Warfarin, which has a long half- life, may be replaced with heparin or low-molecular-weight heparin.

Some drugs are prothrombotic. The oral contraceptive pill should be stopped before major surgery. In general, the risks of thrombosis far outweigh the risks of bleeding and most patients, especially those with additional risk factors, should receive thrombosis prophylaxis if they are having major surgery.

Corticosteroids

The normal basal daily production of cortisol is about 30 mg/day. In response to the stress of surgery this increases to over 100 mg/day. The adrenal gland may be unable to increase steroid production in those who have been taking exogenous steroid medications. There is no consensus about the optimal perioperative steroid supplement regime. A reasonable approach is to give additional steroid cover to those who have been taking oral steroids within 3 months of major surgery. One regime is to give an intravenous loading dose of hydrocortisone (25 mg) followed by an infusion (100 mg) over 24 hours. When a patient who has been taking steroids has unexplained hypotension, an intravenous dose of steroids may be considered.

Table 1 **Perioperative medications**	
Discontinue	**Continue or initiate**
Cardiovascular	
ACE Inhibitors and potassium-sparing diuretics (morning of surgery)	Other antihypertensives
Respiratory	Beta blockers and anti-anginals
	Oxygen
	Asthma medications (preoperative nebulization and steroid cover)
Endocrine	
Long-acting oral hypoglycaemic drugs – convert to insulin sliding scale	Thyroid replacement
	Steroids – additional cover may be required
	Insulin – convert to sliding scale
Neurologic and psychiatric	
Monoamine oxidase inhibitors (2 weeks)	Other psychiatric medications
	Anti-epileptics – add benzodiazepine
Drugs affecting coagulation	
Warfarin – convert to heparin or low-molecular-weight heparin for major surgery	Continue with all anticoagulants where the bleeding risk is low
Oral contraceptive pill and hormone replacement therapy – stop for several weeks	Provide postoperative thrombosis prophylaxis

Clinical case 3

A 38-year-old epileptic woman who had a DVT following previous surgery presents for a cholecystectomy. Her medications include carbamazepine and the oral contraceptive pill. What changes in therapy might be indicated in the perioperative period?
See comments on page 122.

Perioperative medications

- Most therapies should be continued until surgery and restarted immediately thereafter, if necessary via the nasogastric or intravenous route.
- A thorough drug history, including herbal remedies, is essential and if there is doubt the anaesthetist should be consulted about the cessation and continuation of various therapies.
- The more drugs that are administered, the higher the likelihood of an adverse interaction.
- Drug interactions are usually pharmacokinetic (affecting drug levels) or pharmacodynamic (affecting drug action).

Cardiac disease

For patients with cardiac disease, the strain of surgery may result in complications and possible death. Risk-assessment allows medical staff to advise patients appropriately and empowers patients to make informed decisions about their surgery.

- *Coronary artery disease* is the primary risk-factor for postoperative complications. Patients with unstable angina are at risk of myocardial infarction.
- *Cardiomyopathy* carries high morbidity and mortality.
- *Electrical disturbances: atrial fibrillation* increases risk of stroke. *Supraventricular arrhythmias* suggest underlying cardiac disease or metabolic derangements.
- *Valvular heart disease: severe aortic stenosis* carries the risk of sudden death. *Aortic regurgitation* is associated with left ventricular failure with volume overload. *Mitral stenosis* carries the risk of pulmonary congestion, especially with tachycardia. *Mitral regurgitation* is worsened by volume overload. *Mitral valve prolapse* is usually asymptomatic, but in 10% of cases evolves to mitral regurgitation. *Prosthetic valves* increase the risk of endocarditis and thromboembolism.

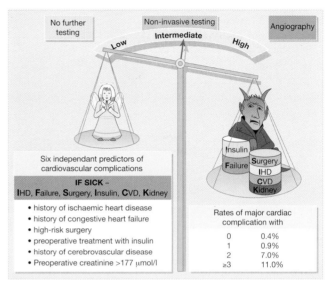

Fig. 1 **Risk-assessment.**

Risk-assessment

Respiratory disease, diabetes mellitus, peripheral vascular disease, systemic hypertension, age, gender, smoking and obesity all modify cardiovascular risk (see Fig. 1).

Risk may be stratified into high, medium, or low risk according to co-existing diseases, level of physical fitness and the extent of the proposed surgery. Patients at highest risk include those with unstable angina, recent myocardial infarction, congestive heart failure, symptomatic arrhythmias and severe valvular heart disease.

Importance of physical fitness

Exercise tolerance is one of the strongest determinants of perioperative risk. Breathlessness or chest pain with minimal exertion augur badly for the ability to tolerate major surgery.

Surgical risk

During certain operations alterations in heart rate, blood pressure, intravascular volume, oxygen carriage and haemoglobin occur. Vascular and thoracic surgery carry particularly high risk. Cardiac complications are 2–5 times more likely following emergency procedures.

Special investigations

Astute clinicians may glean their most useful insights from a targeted history and clinical examination. Special investigations may be superfluous and expensive and may unnecessarily delay surgery. Invasive procedures, like coronary angiography, subject patients to additional risks. Such investigations should be contemplated only when their results may influence management.

Patients falling into the low-risk category may proceed to surgery without further evaluation. The same is applicable to patients having low-risk surgery. Further testing may be most beneficial for patients considered to have intermediate risk. Preoperative cardiac testing is rarely needed if patients have had a coronary evaluation within 2 years or have undergone coronary revascularization within 5 years.

Supplemental preoperative testing aims to:

- Provide an objective measure of exercise tolerance.
- Identify the presence of preoperative myocardial ischaemia.
- Estimate perioperative cardiac risk and assess long-term prognosis.

Non-invasive testing

The resting ECG is not sensitive at detecting ischaemic heart disease.

Exercise ECG is the traditional method of unmasking coronary artery disease (see Fig. 2–3). It is the least invasive and most cost-effective method of detecting ischaemia and determining exercise tolerance.

Unfortunately, exercise ECG is not suitable for all patients. For example those with peripheral vascular disease may be limited in their ability to walk because of claudication. Such patients may have non-exercise (pharmacological) stress testing. Perfusion imaging and stress echocardiography represent appropriate alternatives.

The presence of a redistribution defect on dipyridamole thallium imaging of patients undergoing peripheral vascular surgery is predictive of adverse postoperative cardiac events. Stress echocardiography may reveal regional wall motion abnormalities, which represent areas of myocardium at risk for ischaemic injury. The advantage of this test is that it also provides a dynamic assessment of ventricular function.

Invasive testing

Indications for preoperative coronary angiography are similar to those in the non-surgical setting, including unstable angina or suspected left main or triple-vessel coronary disease.

Arrhythmia control

Many arrhythmias are secondary to metabolic derangements, particularly electrolyte abnormalities. The most common of these abnormalities are hypokalaemia and hypomagnesaemia, which should be corrected well before surgery since the urgent administration of potassium may be hazardous. Pharmacological arrhythmia prophylaxis is of dubious benefit, although there is evidence that amiodarone may decrease the incidence of atrial fibrillation following cardiac surgery.

Coronary reperfusion

As the risks of coronary artery grafting (CAG) frequently exceed the risks of non-cardiac surgery, prophylactic CAG is rarely justified prior to non-cardiac

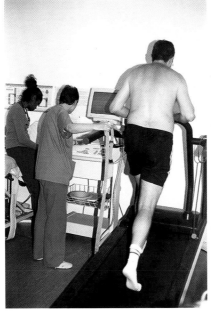

surgery. When long-term and immediate benefit are considered together, the decision to perform a coronary reperfusion procedure prior to a planned elective surgery may be warranted. Occasionally, non-cardiac surgery and CAG may be performed at the same sitting. The role of prophylactic angioplasty and stenting is evolving and may become the technique of choice to decrease risks associated with non-cardiac surgery.

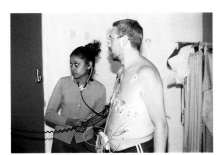

Fig. 2 **Patient undergoing an exercise/ stress ECG.**

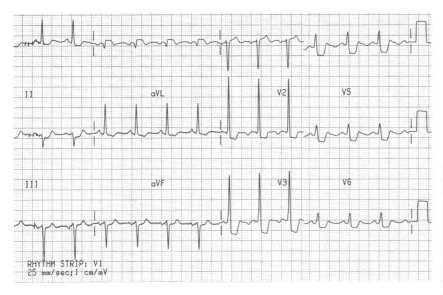

Fig. 3 **Resting ECG showing marked ST depression seen best in anterior and lateral chest leads (V2–V6).** Right axis deviation is also present. Consider severe myocardial ischaemia or posterior MI.

RHYTHM STRIP: V1
25 mm/sec; 1 cm/mV

Clinical case 4

Mr S, a 65-year-old retired teacher, suffers from intermittent claudication after walking 100 metres. He has been admitted electively for a femoral popliteal bypass graft. Mr S does not complain of any chest pain, shortness of breath, swelling of the ankles or palpitations. Does he require further cardiovascular evaluation?
See comments on page 122.

Cardiac disease

- Non-invasive testing should be considered for patients at intermediate risk and those undergoing high-risk surgical procedures.

- Patients at high risk should be considered for angiography, and patients at low risk should not receive further testing.

- Patients with good exercise tolerance have low rates of perioperative cardiac complications.

Hypertension

Hypertension exists when systolic blood pressure is persistently above 140 mmHg or diastolic blood pressure is over 90 mmHg. Symptoms are usually indicative of end-organ damage. The most common causes of death are cerebrovascular and coronary artery disease. Left ventricular hypertrophy, heart failure, renal failure, retinopathy and peripheral vascular disease also occur. Perioperative morbidity and mortality are increased when there is end-organ damage.

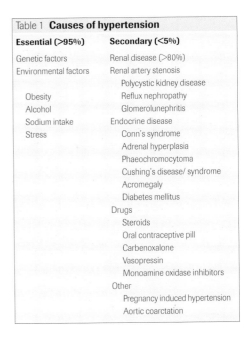

Table 1 **Causes of hypertension**	
Essential (>95%)	**Secondary (<5%)**
Genetic factors	Renal disease (>80%)
Environmental factors	Renal artery stenosis
	Polycystic kidney disease
Obesity	Reflux nephropathy
Alcohol	Glomerolunephritis
Sodium intake	Endocrine disease
Stress	Conn's syndrome
	Adrenal hyperplasia
	Phaeochromocytoma
	Cushing's disease/ syndrome
	Acromegaly
	Diabetes mellitus
	Drugs
	Steroids
	Oral contraceptive pill
	Carbenoxalone
	Vasopressin
	Monoamine oxidase inhibitors
	Other
	Pregnancy induced hypertension
	Aortic coarctation

Causes of hypertension

In 95% of cases, hypertension is essential or without identifiable cause, and is thought to have a multifactorial aetiology (see Table 1). Genetic predispositions are important but environmental factors such as obesity, alcohol and stress also play a role. In the remaining 5% of instances, hypertension is secondary to underlying disease, usually renal or endocrine.

Objectives in evaluating hypertensive patients are:

■ Identification of secondary causes.
■ Assessment of end-organ damage.
■ Quantification of cardiac risk.

Diagnosis

Diagnosing hypertension depends on taking accurate blood pressure readings that reflect the patient's usual resting blood pressure. Readings taken during acute illness or pain should not be used. Single readings may be misleading, as the anxiety of hospital admission may cause temporary hypertension.

The history and examination should focus on symptoms and signs that suggest underlying causes of hypertension or end-organ damage. Markedly elevated blood pressure can cause irreversible end-organ damage and therefore requires urgent attention. The risk of mortality and morbidity rises progressively with increasing systolic and diastolic pressures.

Malignant hypertension is a medical emergency. This diagnosis should be considered with severe hypertension (diastolic blood pressure > 120 mmHg). Elevated blood pressure coupled with flame-shaped haemorrhages, soft exudates or papilloedema on retinal examination is suggestive of malignant hypertension (Fig. 1). Other important findings include proteinuria or haematuria. Irreversible end-organ damage may result if malignant hypertension is left untreated for several hours.

Attention should be paid to the jugular venous pulsation, the presence of left ventricular hypertrophy (Fig. 2) or heart failure and hypertensive retinopathy. Endocrine disease should be excluded and renal masses sought. Neurological examination may reveal previous strokes. The perioperative mortality from undiagnosed phaeochromocytoma, a catecholamine-producing tumour, is at about 50%. Fortunately, this condition is rare and generally causes headaches, palpitations, excessive sweating, labile blood pressure and tachyarrhythmias. The diagnosis is made on the measurement of urinary and plasma catecholamine metabolites.

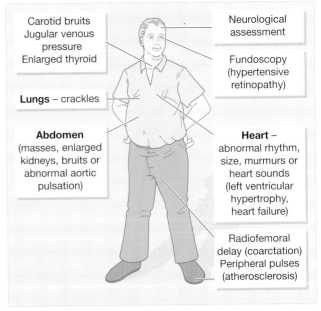

Fig. 1 **Examination of hypertensive patients.**

with diuretic therapy, but may occasionally indicate an underlying endocrine disorder. Aldosterone, cortisol and renin measurements may be made if there is clinical suspicion.

The electrocardiograph (ECG) may display evidence of coronary artery disease or left ventricular hypertrophy. These diagnoses may be pursued with an exercise ECG and echocardiography. The plain chest X-ray may show cardiomegaly or pulmonary congestion if heart failure is developing. Rib-notching on X-ray is suggestive of aortic coarctation, which should be further assessed using magnetic resonance imaging.

Special investigations

Increased creatinine suggests renal impairment, which may be further quantified by means of creatinine clearance, renal ultrasound and renal isotope scans. Low serum K^+ is common

Treatment

Hypertensive patients awaiting elective surgery should be treated and ideally blood pressure should be well controlled for

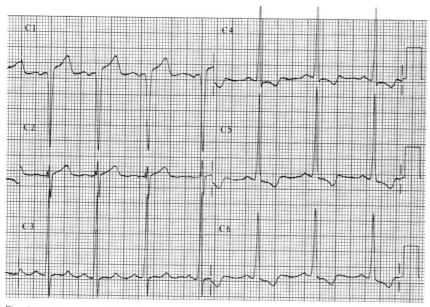

Fig. 2 **ECG trace showing left ventricular hypertrophy with left ventricular strain pattern.**

at least a couple of weeks preceding the operation. Patients with significant hypertension (diastolic pressures > 110 mmHg) should not undergo elective surgery (see Fig. 3). Blood pressure should not be lowered precipitously, but in a controlled manner over several days. The drugs prescribed for hypertension may be modified according to co-existing diseases.

Patients with uncontrolled hypertension have greater intraoperative BP fluctuations than those controlled on treatment. Although hypotension is a more common and feared complication than hypertension, marked increases in systolic blood pressure lasting ≥ 10 minutes increase the risk of myocardial infarction for patients with heart disease.

Fig. 3 **Algorithm for preoperative hypertension.**

Risks of untreated hypertension

Autoregulation of blood flow to the brain, heart, kidneys and liver ensures that perfusion can be maintained even when mean arterial pressures (MAP) is as low as 60 mmHg. However, with chronic untreated hypertension a higher MAP is required to maintain adequate perfusion to vital organs (see Fig. 4). Moderately low BP in a normotensive patient may represent severe hypotension for the hypertensive patient.

Measuring blood pressure

- Caffeine and nicotine should be avoided for 30 minutes prior to measurement.
- Patients should be seated with bare arms supported at heart level (see Fig. 5).
- Use an appropriate cuff size.
- Pressure should be measured after 5 minutes of rest.
- Two or more readings, 2 minutes apart, should be averaged. If readings differ by > 5 mmHg, additional readings are required.

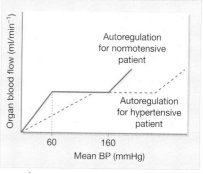

Fig. 4 **Autoregulation of blood flow to vital organs.** In patients with hypertension, perfusion to vital organs is maintained only at higher mean arterial pressures.

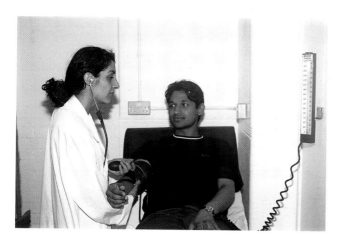

Fig. 5 **Measuring blood pressure.**

Hypertension

- Complications are not increased if preoperative diastolic pressure is below 110 mmHg.
- Hypertension is usually asymptomatic but if left untreated causes end-organ damage.
- Severe hypertension (diastolic > 120 mmHg) may result in perioperative complications, such as myocardial infarction, heart failure, haemorrhagic stroke, encephalopathy and renal failure.
- Patients with uncontrolled hypertension develop marked swings in BP with anaesthesia, blood loss or pain.

Diabetes mellitus

Diabetes mellitus is a persisting state of hyperglycaemia resulting from decreased insulin or diminished efficacy of insulin. Type I diabetes is associated with severe insulin deficiency and Type II diabetes occurs with insulin resistance. Diabetes is the most common endocrine abnormality occurring in all population and age groups.

Diabetes may be controlled by diet, with oral agents, or with insulin. Both Type I and Type II diabetes may require insulin therapy for optimal control. Diabetes has been shown to be an independent risk-factor for vascular disease and sudden cardiac death. Long-term tight control of glucose and blood pressure significantly improves prognosis for diabetics (see Fig. 1). Glycosylated haemoglobin values of 6.5–7.5% probably represent optimal long-term glycaemic control.

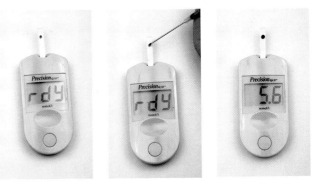

Fig. 1 **Regular use of a glucometer guides dextrose and insulin therapy.**

Effects of diabetes on surgery

In the perioperative period the priority is to avoid the acute life-threatening complications associated with diabetes: hypoglycaemia, diabetic ketoacidosis, and hyperosmolar non-ketotic coma. Control of blood glucose is of benefit in improving wound healing, decreasing infection, and avoiding glycosuria and dehydration.

When plasma glucose levels decrease to about 3.1 mmol/l, the secretion of counter-regulatory hormones increases, and autonomic symptoms (anxiety, palpitations, hunger, sweating, irritability and tremor) appear, as well as neuroglycopaenic symptoms (dizziness, tingling, blurred vision, difficulty in thinking, and faintness). These symptoms, especially the autonomic, induce the correction of hypoglycemia through eating. Some insulin-treated diabetics lose their sensitivity to hypoglycaemia and the plasma glucose concentration must decrease considerably before the counter-regulatory response and symptoms occur. The sedated patient in the perioperative period is at heightened risk of life-threatening hypoglycaemia. Particular attention should also be paid to patients taking beta-blockers as these medications mask the symptoms of hypoglycaemia.

Nature of surgery

Those with diabetes present for all types of surgery, but the disease process itself increases the likelihood of certain operations, including cardiac, vascular and eye surgery. A disproportionate number of patients undergoing abscess drainage and septic debridement have diabetes, as there is a strong association between diabetes and infection.

Tight control

While it is imperative to ensure that life-threatening hypoglycaemia does not occur, in certain patients, tight control of blood glucose (3.5–6 mmo/l) is particularly important (see Fig. 2). This applies to any patient who may be at risk of ischaemic nervous system injury. Under anaerobic conditions, glucose is metabolised to lactate, which may worsen acidosis in nervous tissue. This applies to patients with head injuries, following cardiac arrest, those having cardiac or neurosurgery, and any patient with circulatory shock. Tight control of maternal blood glucose throughout pregnancy and labour improves the outcome for mother and baby.

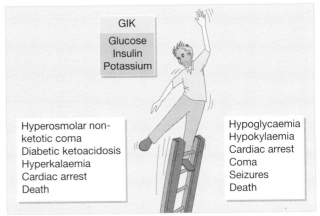

Fig. 2 **Tight control is like walking a tightrope. Glucose, insulin and potassium must be tightly controlled and balanced to avoid hazards.**

Effects of surgery on diabetes

Patients with diabetes are at increased risk for complications in the perioperative period. When they are drowsy or sedated, they are unable to communicate symptoms of hypo- or hyperglycaemia and are unable to take responsibility for the control of their own blood sugar levels. Several factors heighten risk. Patients are fasted prior to surgery, rendering them vulnerable to hypoglycaemia. Insulin therapy and oral sulphonylureas taken without food compound the problem. Surgery is a potent activator of the stress response and the stress hormones (adrenaline, cortisol, growth hormone and thyroid hormone) all oppose the actions of insulin, thus promoting hyperglycaemia. If vigilance decreases following surgery diabetic ketoacidosis may occur (see Fig. 3).

Co-existing diseases

Diabetes is associated with several disease processes and it is important to consider both diseases which impact on postoperative outcome and diseases which may be exacerbated by surgery (Table 1). Therapeutic options for painful peripheral neuropathy include tricyclic

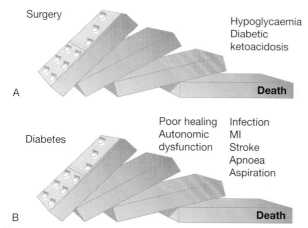

Fig. 3 **(a) Possible effects of surgery on diabetes. (b) Possible effects of diabetes on surgery.**

Table 2 **Sample sliding scale**	
4-hourly blood glucose	**Action**
0–3.5 mmol/l	Start 500 ml 5% dextrose iv and call doctor
3.5–8 mmol/l	None
8–10 mmol/l	2 units soluble insulin iv or S/C
10–14 mmol/l	4 units insulin
14–16 mmol/l	6 units insulin
16–18 mmol/l	8 units insulin
>18 mmol/l	10 units insulin and call doctor

Diabetics should be first on operating lists and, postoperatively should be encouraged to eat and resume control of their blood sugar as soon as possible.

Diabetic ketoacidosis

Diabetic ketoacidosis (DKA) is a medical emergency, which may be precipitated by surgery, infection, myocardial infarction and trauma. All of these insults may occur in the perioperative period. Transfer to ICU is recommended.

Treatment of DKA

- Soluble insulin by infusion. The initial rate is 6 units per hour. This may be increased incrementally if blood sugar does not decrease. Insulin should be continued until metabolic acidosis, hyperglycaemia, and ketonuria have all resolved.
- Fluids. There is a deficit of up to 12 litres, but over-zealous replacement may cause cerebral oedema. Administer normal saline until blood glucose is less than 15 mmol/l. Thereafter use 5% dextrose.
- Potassium. Even with high potassium in the blood, there is intracellular potassium depletion, with a usual deficit of 3–10 mmol/kg. When the insulin is started patients usually require up to 20–40 mmol/hour of potassium.
- Supportive. This includes oxygen and treatment of possible precipitating causes. Phosphorous and magnesium may be required. Acidosis usually responds to fluids and insulin, but bicarbonate may be indicated as a temporizing measure if the pH is less than 7.

Table 1 **Diabetes and co-existing disease**		
Disease process	**Risk in perioperative period**	**Important considerations**
Autonomic neuropathy	Delayed gastric emptying – aspiration	Antacid and prokinetic premedication
	Painless myocardial ischaemia – silent infarction	Investigate for coronary artery disease
	Apnoea	Supplementary oxygen and monitor breathing
Peripheral neuropathy	Pressure necrosis	Protect pressure points
	Increased sensitivity to local anaesthetics	Document neuropathies and decrease local anaesthetic dosage
Vascular disease	Acute vascular events – MI, CVA	Maintain coronary, renal and cerebral perfusion pressure
Nephropathy	Acute renal failure	Maintain intravascular volume
		Osmotic diuresis may occur with hyperglycaemia
		Avoid nephrotoxic drugs
Immunocompromised	Infection	Antibiotic prophylaxis and treat infection
Stiff joints including cervical spine	Difficult intubation and airway management	Avoidance of general anaesthesia if possible

antidepressants, phenytoin, carbamazepine and topical capsaicin. Diabetic gastroparesis may improve with metoclopramide or erythromycin.

Perioperative management

Elective surgery should only be performed when diabetes is well controlled. Patients having minor surgery and day-case surgery may continue with their therapy. Blood glucose should be checked preoperatively. Those having major surgery should be admitted the day before surgery and should probably have their oral treatment converted to an insulin sliding scale (Table 2).

Preoperative fasting is important in view of a possible delay in gastric emptying. A 5% dextrose infusion should be commenced to prevent hypoglycaemia and to provide nutrition. It is an important concept that while diabetics may have high glucose in their blood, their cells are frequently undernourished, as they are unable to utilize the glucose.

Clinical case 5

On the morning that he is scheduled for surgery, a patient who has diabetes is fitting on the ward. He has no other diseases and was previously well. What should be done?
See comment on page 122.

Diabetes mellitus

- The priority is to prevent hypoglycaemia, diabetic ketoacidosis, and hyperosmolar non-ketotic coma.
- The sedated patient is at heightened risk of life-threatening hypoglycaemia.
- Diabetes worsens surgical outcome and surgery may precipitate complications associated with diabetes.
- Diabetics should be first on operating lists.

Thrombophilia and bleeding tendency

The coagulation system has been under considerable evolutionary pressure because it balances the risks of haemorrhage against those of thrombosis (Fig. 1). Never are these risks as delicately poised as in the perioperative period. Bleeding is an obvious risk associated with surgery. Deep venous thrombosis (DVT) and pulmonary embolism (PE) are common causes of in-hospital morbidity and mortality.

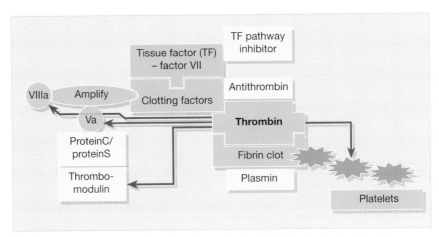

Fig. 1 **Simplified depiction of clotting (green) and anticlotting (yellow) pathways.**

Thrombophilia

Thrombophilia is an abnormal tendency for the blood to clot. The clot can be either in an artery or a vein. Arterial thromboses (AT) are potentially more serious, but venous thromboses . The incidence of DVTs following major orthopaedic surgery exceeds 50%. Minimizing risk-factors and preventing thrombosis are important aspects of perioperative care.

Causes

A patient might develop a thrombus due to a variety of predisposing factors (Table 1). Recognition of the patients at risk and early liaison with a haematologist are key to a successful outcome. Virchow's triad (Fig. 2) describes three important prothrombotic conditions, all of which occur during surgery.

Prophylaxis

Stop combined oral contraceptives 4 weeks before major surgery and all leg surgery. For elective surgery, encourage patients to lose weight and stop smoking. Regional rather than general anaesthesia should be considered. Calf compression devices, elastic stockings, physiotherapy and early mobilization are indicated postoperatively (Fig. 3). For many patients, the above conservative measures are insufficient

and anticoagulant medications are required.

Heparin

Heparin opposes clotting by potentiating the action of antithrombin. The two types of heparin in use are unfractionated heparin, which has a short half-life, and low-molecular-weight heparin (LMWH), which has a longer duration of action. Both types are currently recommended for thrombosis prophylaxis in patients at risk, but LWMH may be more effective especially in orthopaedic practice.

Warfarin

The INR (international normalized ratio) is a marker of warfarin's therapeutic effect. The INR should be < 1.5 for major surgery. Medication should be switched from warfarin to heparin 3–4 days prior to major surgery. When warfarin is restarted, onset of anticoagulation takes 48–72 hours. So heparin or LMWH should be administered concurrently.

Reversal of anticoagulation

If surgery is elective, there is time to rationalize anticoagulation therapy. For emergency surgery, subcutaneous vitamin K 1 mg will rapidly normalize

an elevated INR due to warfarin, and protamine is the reversal drug for heparin. Anticoagulation should be restarted as soon as safety allows. Table 2 shows suggested perioperative management of anticoagulation in those at high risk.

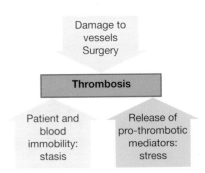

Fig. 2 **Virchow's triad.**

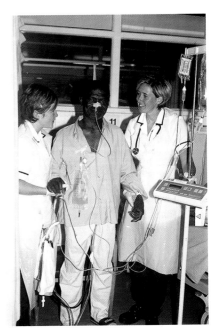

Fig. 3 **A patient walking early to prevent venous thrombosis.**

Table 1 **Risk-factors for thrombosis**		
Congenital	**Acquired**	**Precipitating**
Protein S or C deficiency	Malignancy	Obesity (BMI > 30 kg/m²)
Activated protein C resistance (factor V Leiden)	Antiphospholipid syndrome	Pregnancy
		Oral contraceptive pill
Abnormality of fibrinogen		
Abnormality or deficiency of antithrombin III		Immobility and bed-rest
Prothrombin 20210		Smoking
Increased factor XI, IX, VIII		Surgery, especially pelvic and orthopaedic

Table 2 **Perioperative management of anticoagulation in high-risk patients**		
Indication	Preoperative	Postoperative
< 1 month after DVT	Full heparinization[1] or vena caval filter	Full heparinization
2–3 months post DVT	S/C heparin[2] or LMWH[3]	Full heparinization
History of recurrent DVT	S/C heparin or LMWH	S/C heparin or LMWH
< 1 month post arterial embolism	Full heparinization	Full heparinization
Mechanical heart valve	S/C heparin or LMWH	S/C heparin or LMWH
Nonvalvular atrial fibrillation	S/C heparin or LMWH	S/C heparin or LMWH

[1], unfraction heparin 1–2000 units per hour i.v. (adjust according to APTT); [2], unfractionated heparin 5000 units S/C energy 8–10 hours; [3], enoxaparin 40 mg S/C daily

Bleeding tendecies

Bleeding tendencies may result from dysfunction in the clotting cascade (for example haemophilia A), platelet insufficiency or malfunction, hypothermia, anticoagulant medications, consumption of platelets and clotting factors, or following major blood loss (Fig. 4). As with thrombophilia, advice from a haematologist should be sought. Management of postoperative bleeding is considered on pages 70–71.

Von Willebrand's disease

von Willebrand's Disease (vWD) is the most common inherited bleeding diathesis, with an estimated 1% of the population having a form of the disorder. The defect is in von Willebrand factor (vWF), required for platelet adhesiveness and as a carrier for factor VIII. There are three types of vWD and perioperative management depends on the type.

Blood products, including cryoprecipitate, fresh frozen plasma FVIII (recombinant or concentrate), desmopressin, and platelets, have been used to treat vWD. Bleeding time and laboratory clotting tests may provide information about bleeding tendency. Platelet aggregometry yields more definitive picture about severity.

Factor deficiencies

Haemophilia, a lack of factor VIII (FVIII), is the most common clotting factor deficiency. It is an X-linked condition, so typically males are affected. Females may carry the gene and be mildly affected. The relative lack of FVIII varies from patient to patient. Serious bleeding is rare when FVIII levels are above 5% of normal, but for surgical purposes more than 50% is desirable. FVIII is given at the time of surgery to achieve adequate levels.

Christmas disease (FIX deficiency) is also X-linked, and is treated with once-daily FIX infusions to maintain normal levels after surgery. Deficiencies in other clotting factors can also cause significant bleeding and treatment is usually by replacement of the relevant factor.

Patients with clotting deficiencies should not be given I.M. injections. Intramuscular bleeding and compression damage may result.

Platelet disorders

Decreased platelet number and disorders of platelet function can lead to bleeding tendencies. Platelet number in excess of 50×10^9 per litre is usually sufficient for normal haemostasis. Platelet transfusion prior to major surgery should be considered.

Management

Patients with a personal or family history of excessive bleeding (easy bruising, bleeding gums or epistaxes) might have a bleeding disorder that warrants investigation. Even minor bleeding disorders can radically affect surgical procedures. Although minor surgery is unlikely to result in serious blood loss, in some types of operations, such as ophthalmic and neurological surgery, even small bleeds can have devastating results.

Whereas in thrombophilia regional anaesthesia might be advantageous, with a bleeding disorder it could be disastrous. Bleeding following spinal or epidural anaesthesia can result in haematoma formation that compresses the spinal cord and causes permanent neurological deficit. Fortunately this is a rare complication. Haematoma usually causes backache and this complaint should not be ignored. Regional anaesthesia should be avoided when a bleeding tendancy is suspected.

Clinical case 6

A 51-year-old woman has carcinoma of the stomach. She presented with lethargy and breathlessness, which were due to recurrent DVTs and pulmonary emboli. She has been taking warfarin for 6 weeks. In one week, she is scheduled to undergo surgery for tumour resection. Her current INR is 4. How should she be managed perioperatively in terms of her risks for bleeding and clotting?
See comment on page 122.

Thrombophilia and bleeding tendency

- Thrombophilia is more common than bleeding tendencies.
- Early liaison with a haemotologist is important.
- Patients at risk of thrombophilia should be identified before surgery, and their risk-factors managed accordingly.
- Patients having major surgery should generally receive thrombosis prophylaxis.

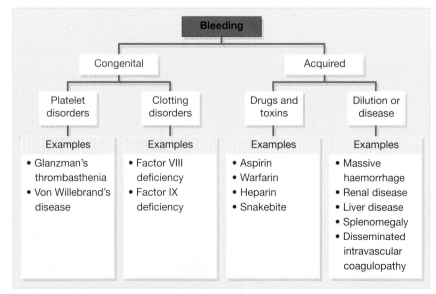

Fig. 4 **Classification of bleeding tendencies.**

Obesity

Obesity is the most common nutritional disorder in the developed world. Recent figures estimate that 8% of males and 12% of females in the UK are obese. In the USA obesity is said to affect up to 33% of the population. Obesity is a potent risk-factor for many conditions including coronary heart disease, hypertension and non-insulin dependent diabetes mellitus, all of which contribute independently to increased risk of postoperative morbidity and mortality. Weight loss may not only help control diseases worsened by obesity, it may also help decrease the likelihood of developing these diseases. Excess fat in the neck and jaw renders obese patients prone to upper airway obstruction.

Indices of obesity

The most widely used indicator of obesity is the body mass index (BMI), which is weight (kg)/height (m²). The risk of coronary heart disease is doubled if the BMI exceeds 25 kg/m² and is almost quadrupled when the index is above 29 kg/m². People with a BMI over 35 kg/m² have a 40-fold increased chance of developing type II diabetes mellitus.

The BMI, however, fails to provide any information regarding fat distribution, which itself has an important association with the development of cardiovascular disease. Abdominal fat is associated with insulin resistance, hyperinsulinaemia and high blood pressure. Apart from impaired glucose tolerance, there is increased frequency of diabetes mellitus and hyperlipidaemia resulting in atheroma formation. As adipose cells increase in size and number they are thought to bind high-density lipoprotein (HDL), thereby lowering the blood levels and decreasing the protection afforded against the formation of atheromatous plaques.

Abdominal obesity occurs more commonly in males where fat is localized to the trunk, giving rise to an apple shape, whereas premenopausal females tend to store fat around the hips, the healthier pear shape. Abdominal fat can be evaluated simply with the waist to hip ratio (WHR). This is the waist circumference (cm)/hip circumference (cm). In women, the risk of cardiovascular disease is increased if the WHR is > 0.8 and for men if it is > 1.

Obesity and co-existing disease

Obesity is associated with a number of medical conditions, the most notable being an increase in cardiovascular disease and respiratory abnormalities (Table 1).

Hypertension

In overweight young adults aged 20–45, the prevalence of hypertension is six times that of their normal-weight peers. The distribution of fat in the body may have an important effect on blood-pressure risk (see Fig. 1), with central or upper body fat being more likely to raise blood pressure than lower body fat.

Diabetes

Even moderate obesity, particularly abdominal obesity, can increase the risk of type II diabetes mellitus. Weight reduction leads to improvement of glycaemic control as well as improvement of other medical problems such as hypertension or hyperlipidaemia.

Pulmonary abnormalities

There are several abnormalities in pulmonary function in obese individuals. At one extreme are patients with Pickwickian syndrome, or the obesity–hypoventilation syndrome, which is characterized by somnolence and hypoventilation, and eventually cor pulmonale.

In patients who are less obese, there is a fairly uniform decrease in expiratory reserve volume and a tendency to reduction in all lung volumes. A low maximum rate of voluntary ventilation and venous admixture are also present. As an individual becomes more obese, the muscular work required for ventilation increases. In addition, respiratory muscles may not function normally in obese individuals.

Obstructive sleep apnoea

Obstructive sleep apnoea syndrome or Pickwickian syndrome is defined as a 10-second apnoea occurring at least thirty times during sleep. In most cases it is caused by upper airway obstruction secondary to excess fat in the neck and jaw. Increased fat in the chest wall and abdomen decrease chest wall compliance and residual

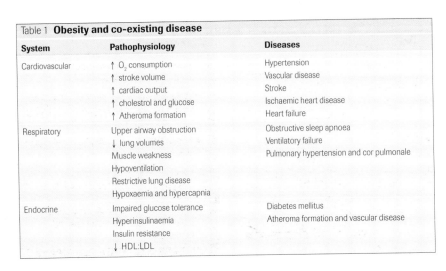

Table 1 Obesity and co-existing disease		
System	**Pathophysiology**	**Diseases**
Cardiovascular	↑ O₂ consumption	Hypertension
	↑ stroke volume	Vascular disease
	↑ cardiac output	Stroke
	↑ cholestrol and glucose	Ischaemic heart disease
	↑ Atheroma formation	Heart failure
Respiratory	Upper airway obstruction	Obstructive sleep apnoea
	↓ lung volumes	Ventilatory failure
	Muscle weakness	Pulmonary hypertension and cor pulmonale
	Hypoventilation	
	Restrictive lung disease	
	Hypoxaemia and hypercapnia	
Endocrine	Impaired glucose tolerance	Diabetes mellitus
	Hyperinsulinaemia	Atheroma formation and vascular disease
	Insulin resistance	
	↓ HDL:LDL	

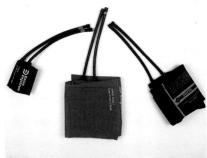

Fig. 1 ·**Different blood pressure cuff sizes.**

lung volumes. Small airway closure combined with increased O_2 consumption renders obese people susceptible to episodes of low oxygen saturation. Clinical manifestations of the syndrome vary according to severity, and include lethargy, somnolence and loss of central responsiveness to CO_2. A sleep study can confirm the diagnosis (see Fig. 2).

Gastrointestinal

There is an increased incidence of gastro-oesophageal reflux and hiatus hernia. These factors, coupled with increased abdominal pressure render obese individuals susceptible to aspiration of gastric contents.

Pharmacological considerations

Increased fat stores and volume of distribution may prolong the elimination half-life of lipid-soluble drugs. Intramuscular injections are best avoided, as there is unpredictable absorption from fatty tissue. Most drugs do not penetrate fat as readily as well-perfused tissue groups. It is therefore easy to give these patients overdoses. Dosing should be calculated according to lean body mass, and opioids in particular should be given with caution, bearing in mind the hazards of even mild ventilatory depression. Medications to reduce gastric acidity and to promote stomach emptying are appropriate.

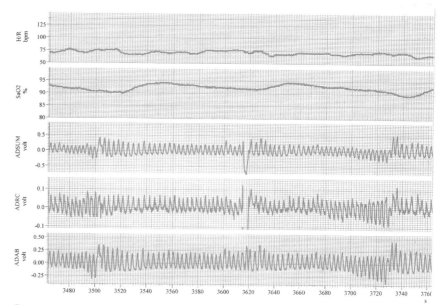

Fig. 2 **Trace showing heart rate, oxygen saturation and respiratory muscle activity during sleep study.**

Postoperative care

In the initial postoperative period, care in a high dependency unit is advisable. Episodes of hypoxaemia are common and may precipitate other complications, like myocardial ischaemia, pulmonary hypertension, and cardiac arrhythmias. Oxygen should be administered for up to 3 days postoperatively and continuous positive airway pressure may be useful during sleep.

A pulse oximeter will alert staff if there is prolonged hypoxaemia. Arterial blood gases reveal carbon dioxide retention and worsening lung function.

Patients should be nursed in a semi recumbent position and regular chest physiotherapy may prevent pulmonary atelectasis. Patient-controlled analgesia is preferred to regular opioid injections as it achieves satisfactory pain-relief with less respiratory depression. Early mobilization and other measures are important to prevent venous thrombosis in this high-risk group.

> ### Clinical case 7
>
> A 45-year-old woman is scheduled for gallbladder surgery. She weighs 130 kg and is 150 cm tall. Her abdominal girth is 120 cm and her hip circumference is 130 cm. Blood pressure is 140/90 mmHg, pulse is 75/min and respiration is 10 breaths/min. She has no known medical problems. Calculate and comment on her indices of obesity.
> *See comment on page 122.*

> ### Obesity
>
> ■ Obesity is associated with increased morbidity and mortality.
>
> ■ Preoperative assessment should focus on improving fitness for surgery and planning perioperative management.
>
> ■ Regional anaesthesia may be preferable to general anaesthesia.
>
> ■ Patients are at increased risk for postoperative complications including airway obstruction, hypoxaemia, chest infection, venous thrombosis, wound infection, cardiac complications and pulmonary embolus.

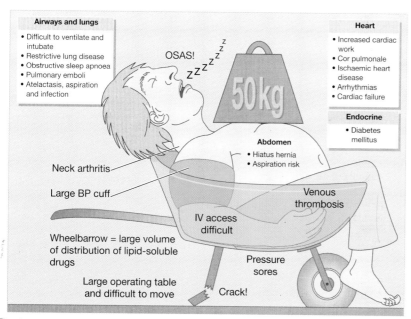

Fig. 3 **Perioperative considerations in obese individuals.**

Pulmonary disease

Cardiac and respiratory complications account for the major slice of postoperative morbidity. The priorities are to identify those at risk and where possible to decrease risk before surgery, to use the safest surgical and anaesthetic techniques and to employ strategies aimed at preventing postoperative pulmonary compromise.

Assessment of lung function

Simple assessment of exercise tolerance is the most cost-effective and possibly the best predictor of postoperative pulmonary function. Abnormalities detected in clinical examination, including dullness to percussion and abnormal breath sounds, have also been correlated with pulmonary complications.

The chest X-ray may provide valuable information; asymptomatic malignancy for example may be revealed on a plain X-ray (Fig. 1)

Asthma is best evaluated by longitudinal testing with a peak flowmeter, rather than with one-off tests of lung function. Spirometry findings are not predictive of pulmonary complications, but may be useful in detecting whether those with asthma or obstructive airways disease have a reversible component, which would improve with therapy. Arterial blood gases provide information about the severity of lung disease, but have not been demonstrated to predict the need for postoperative ventilation.

Smoking

It is not surprising that pulmonary disease is prevalent in the UK given that 25% of adults smoke. All smokers suffer untoward effects, the extent of which depends on amount smoked, genetic factors and luck. Smokers have hyper-reactive airways, rendering them more vulnerable to laryngospasm and bonchospasm. Ciliary function is compromised and the ability to clear secretions is impaired, both of which contribute to increased susceptibility to respiratory tract infections. Surprisingly, cessation of smoking preoperatively initially increases the incidence of postoperative infection, peaking at about 2 weeks. The risk decreases to baseline levels at between 4–8 weeks and major benefit is only realised after 2–3 months (Fig. 2).

Nicotine and carbon monoxide (CO) are constituents of cigarette smoke. CO binds to haemoglobin (Hb) with a greater affinity than oxygen does and smokers have up to 10% of Hb as carboxyhaemoglobin. For those with borderline oxygen carrying capacity, this amount may be critical. The graph illustrates the left shift in the oxygen dissociation graph that occurs with CO, rendering haemoglobin less capable of offloading its oxygen carriage (Fig. 3). Cigarettes are inducers of hepatic enzymes and smokers may require higher dosages of drugs which undergo liver metabolism. Nicotine causes tachycardia, arrhythmias and CNS stimulation (see Table 1). Nicotine deprivation precipitates an acute withdrawal syndrome. Smokers are advised to quit smoking before surgery for at least 2 months.

Chronic bronchitis, obstructive airways disease, peripheral and coronary vascular disease sequelae of long-term smoking. Smoking is also a risk-factor for various malignancies, including lung and upper-airway cancers. The morbidity associated with

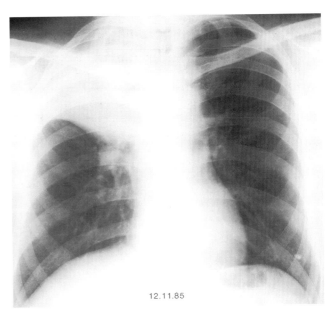

12.11.85

Fig. 1 **Chest X-ray showing suspicious lesion in the lung field, which may be a malignancy.**

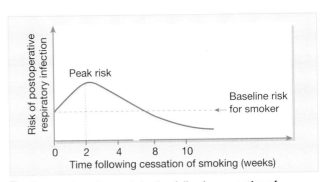

Fig. 2 **Risk of respiratory infection following cessation of smoking.**

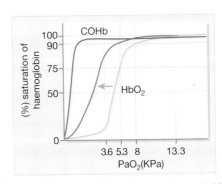

Fig. 3 **Effect of carbon monoxide on the oxyhaemoglobin dissociation curve.**

Table 1 **The effects of smoking**		
Tobacco chemical	**Effect**	**Disease associations**
Nicotine	Increased heart rate, blood pressure and cardiac output	Hypertension, coronary heart disease, stroke
Tar	Damages cilia and alveoli	Lung, mouth, pharynx, trachea, larynx cancers
CO	Binds to Hb, makes CO-Hb, decreases O_2-Hb	Coronary heart disease, stroke

smoking relates to pack years (Fig. 4). A pack year is the equivalent of smoking 20 cigarettes-a-day for a year (or 10-a-day for 2 years or 40-a-day for 6 months).

Chronic obstructive pulmonary disease

There is a spectrum of disease from chronic bronchitis to emphysema. Most sufferers are smokers or ex-smokers. If surgery is deemed essential in patients with these disorders, several strategies can be adopted to improve outcome. In the preoperative period, reversible problems may be identified and treated so that health is optimal when patients present for surgery (see Table 2).

Both surgical and anaesthetic technique should be tailored to minimizing pulmonary impairment. Methods of decreasing postoperative complications are covered on page 66. Teaching

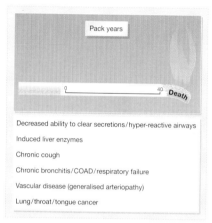

Decreased ability to clear secretions/hyper-reactive airways

Induced liver enzymes

Chronic cough

Chronic bronchitis/COAD/respiratory failure

Vascular disease (generalised arteriopathy)

Lung/throat/tongue cancer

Fig. 4 **Timeline associated with pack years of smoking.**

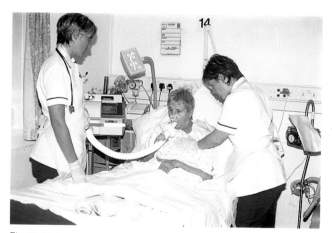

Fig. 5 **Patient using a spirometer.**

patients incentive spirometry and deep-breathing exercises improves postoperative lung function. Preoperative admission to a medical ward for optimization may be a worthwhile consideration. Thrombosis prophylaxis is indicated.

Asthma

Asthma is a reactive airways disease, in which a varying degree of reversible bronchospasm is the presenting feature. Severity of disease may be difficult to gauge because, during asymptomatic periods, physical examination is normal. History provides crucial information in the preoperative assessment. Severity of asthma may be ascertained from serial peak flow measurements, information about the impact of the disease on normal activities and a history of hospital or intensive care admissions.

The drug therapy required to control asthma also provides valuable insights. If bronchodilator therapy improves lung function as measured by spirometry (see Fig. 5), then 2 weeks of steroid therapy (1–2 mg/kg p.o. prednisolone) is advisable prior to surgery. For elective surgery, the peak flow should be greater than 80% of the predicted normal or the patient's best value, and there should be no wheezing on chest examination.

Manipulation of the airway may precipitate bronchospasm, and tracheal intubation is best avoided. Many drugs induce histamine release, and alternatives are advisable.

Other lung diseases

Many diseases affect the lungs. The respiratory tract is the most common portal for infection. Multi-drug-resistant tuberculosis is on the increase. The human immunodeficiency virus pandemic is accompanied by a variety of pulmonary infections. Various occupations, like mining and farming, place workers at risk for occupational lung disease. There are congenital diseases, like cystic fibrosis and alpha-1 antitrypsin deficiency, which have important pulmonary manifestations. Several multisystem disorders including sarcoidosis, rheumatoid arthritis and systemic lupus erythematosis have pulmonary components. Failure of other organs, like the heart, liver and kidneys has adverse consequences for the lungs. Specialist advice on the management of such patients should be sought prior to surgery.

Clinical case 8

An asymptomatic asthmatic woman presents for an elective hernia operation. Physical examination is normal. Peak flow is 70% of predicted and significantly less than she achieved 2 weeks ago at the general practitioner. Is she fit for surgery?
See comment on page 122.

Pulmonary disease

■ Exercise tolerance is the best predictor of postoperative pulmonary function.

■ Smoking is associated with a high incidence of lung disease.

■ At least 8 weeks' cessation of smoking is required before there is a positive impact on postoperative complications.

■ Asthma and COPD must be optimally controlled before elective surgery.

Table 2 **Treatable complications of chronic obstructive disease pulmonary (COPD)**	
Complication	**Treatment**
Chest infection	Appropriate antibiotics and chest physiotherapy
Bronchospasm	Two weeks of steroid therapy and perioperative nebulised ipratroprium and B_2 agonist
Cor pulmonale	Judicious use of diuretic therapy. Oxygen to treat pulmonary hypertension. Admission to medical ward for preoperative optimization
Respiratory failure	Oxygen therapy and breathing exercises. Theophylline may be of some value
Polycythaemia (increased haemoglobin)	Venesection. Blood obtained may be used for autologous transfusion during surgery
Decreased effort tolerance	Exercise

HIV and other viruses

Viruses can be transmitted through exposure to blood and blood products. The most important of these are: human immunodeficiency virus (HIV), hepatitis B virus (HBV) and hepatitis C virus (HCV).

Transmission

Transmission of HBV, HCV and HIV is:

- Vertical – mother to baby (including breast feeding).
- Horizontal – through sexual intercourse or through inoculation of blood/blood products.

The risk of transmission from a single infectious needle-stick injury is estimated as 30% for HBV, 3% for HCV and 0.3% for HIV.

Hepatitis B virus

The major antigens of HBV are surface antigen (HBsAg), Core antigen (HBcAg) and secreted protein (HBeAg) (Fig. 1). HBV has an incubation period of 2–6 months, which is followed by acute hepatitis. Jaundice may not be apparent in 50%. Fulminant hepatitis and liver failure occur in less than 1%. Chronic infection occurs in 5%. If HBsAg remains seropositive for more than 6 months, then persistent infection (carrier status) is diagnosed. Carriers are infectious to others and particularly so if HBeAg is also seropositive.

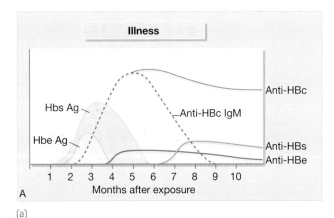

(a)

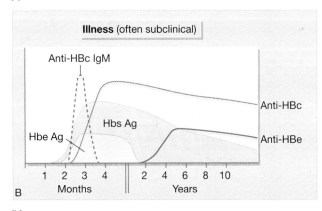

(b)

Fig. 1 **(a) Serology of acute HBV infection. (b) Serology of chronic HBV infection.**

HBV vaccination is essential for healthcare workers. Healthcare workers are not permitted to carry out invasive procedures or operations if they are HBeAg positive (high-risk) carriers of HBV. Hyperimmune hepatitis B immunoglobulin (HBIG) and vaccination can be administered after accidental exposure to infected blood or body fluids in an unvaccinated individual. Interferon-alpha and lamivudine are efficacious in the treatment of chronic HBV.

Human immunodeficiency virus

The human retroviruses, HIV 1 and HIV 2, infect CD4-carrying cells.

The incubation period of HIV is 3–6 weeks, after which there is an acute seroconversion illness followed by an asymptomatic phase of 2–10 years. There is persistent viral replication and progressive decline in CD4-T cell levels. The onset of AIDS occurs with the development of -opportunistic infections or when the CD4T cells have declined below 200 cells/mm³.

Antiretroviral therapy (ART) greatly improves the prognosis of HIV infection and is given in combinations of three or more drugs from the classes of nucleoside analogues, non-nucleoside reverse transcriptase inhibitors and protease inhibitors.

Post-exposure prophylaxis of triple antiretroviral therapy can be offered to healthcare workers after accidental exposure to HIV. This therapy, consisting of agents such as lamivudine, zidovudine and indinavir, should be taken as soon as possible after the accident, preferably within a few hours, and continued for 4 weeks. Packs of emergency ART are usually kept in the hospital Accident and Emergency or Pharmacy departments. There is currently no effective vaccine available against HIV.

Hepatitis C virus

Hepatitis C virus has been sequenced from the serum of sufferers and visualized with electron microscopy, but has not been cultured. Following infection, usually as a result of inoculation of blood or body fluids, there is an incubation period of 3–10 weeks.

Only about 5% of patients become jaundiced and chronic infection develops in about 80%. Chronic liver damage with cirrhosis and hepatocellular carcinoma occurs after 10–15 years in a minority. Persistent mild hepatitis, manifesting biochemically as raised transaminases, can persist for decades.

Patients with chronic infection remain potentially infectious to others. Antibodies to HCV and viral RNA, detected by PCR, can be demonstrated in the serum. Ribavirin and interferon-alpha are used in the treatment of chronic HCV. There is no vaccine available.

Prevention of transmission in the hospital setting

Every patient should be regarded as potentially infected with a blood-borne virus. Precautions are therefore universally implemented (summarized in Tables 1 and 2, see Fig. 2).

The acronym 'ASSAULT' is a useful memory aid for the safe handling of sharps within the healthcare setting:

- Attention to
- Safety and
- Sharps policy
- Accident reporting
- Universal precautions
- Labelling of specimens correctly
- Transport of specimens safely.

Following an injury

- Follow local policy
- Wash site of injury thoroughly with soap and water.

- Irrigate mucous membrane splash with plenty of water.
- Discuss the necessity for ART with designated infectious disease or virology physician
- Report to occupational health.

Table 1 **Universal precautions**	
Precaution	**Comments**
Hand washing	Before and after examinations and procedures
Protective clothing	Gloves, gowns, goggles and face visor
Disposal of waste	Infected waste should be incinerated
Disposal of sharps	No resheathing of needles, disposal in a sharps bin close to the patient, no re-use of disposables
Spills	Blood should be cleared up with hypochlorite solution
Accident reporting	To the occupational health department

Table 2 **Categorization of body fluids according to the risk of transmission of blood-borne virus infections**	
High-risk body fluids	**Low-risk body fluids**
Blood	Faeces
Body fluid visibly stained with blood	Nasal secretions
Cerebrospinal fluid	Sputum
Peritoneal fluid	Sweat
Pleural fluid	Tears
Pericardial fluid	Urine
Synovial fluid	Vomit
Amniotic fluid	Saliva (except in dentistry)
Semen	
Vaginal secretions	
Saliva in the context of dentistry	

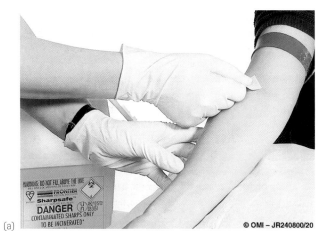
(a) © OMI – JR240800/20

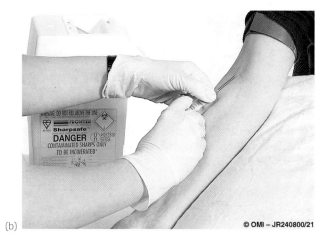
(b) © OMI – JR240800/21

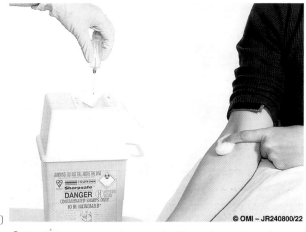
(c) © OMI – JR240800/22

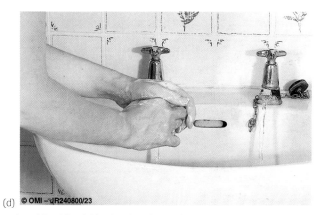
(d) © OMI – JR240800/23

Fig. 2 **(a–d) Sequence of photographs illustrating universal precautions in taking blood.** Note hand washing before and after the procedure, wearing of gloves, use of the vacutainer® system and the immediate safe disposal of the contaminated sharp.

Clinical case 9

During the drug round, while performing a deep intramuscular injection, a nurse stabs himself in the hand. What should he do?
See comment on page 122.

HIV and other viruses

- Universal precautions should be adhered to.
- Re-use of disposable equipment or potentially contaminated equipment is unacceptable practice.
- Healthcare workers should be vaccinated against HBV.
- Early post-exposure antiretroviral prophylaxis decreases the chance of HIV infection.

Alcohol and substance abuse

Substance abuse is on the increase in many societies. Long-term drug usage results in organ damage. Chronic alcohol abuse, for example, is related to a number of medical complications including liver damage, cardiomyopathy and peptic ulceration. Substance abusers have a higher incidence of perioperative morbidity and mortality and therefore require careful management.

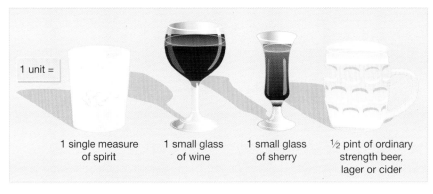

Fig. 1 **One unit of alcohol.**

1 unit =

1 single measure of spirit

1 small glass of wine

1 small glass of sherry

½ pint of ordinary strength beer, lager or cider

Alcohol (ethanol)

Almost all adults in the UK drink and alcohol consumption is a societal norm. Alcohol is a cerebral depressant, which is thought to mediate its effects through GABA stimulation. It has potent anxiolytic effects producing disinhibition and relaxation in small amounts.

The recommended maximum alcohol volumes are 21 units per week for men and 14 units per week for women. One unit equates to 8 g of ethanol, which is equivalent to a half-pint of beer, one glass of wine or a single measure of spirits (Fig. 1). One definition of alcohol abuse is consumption of 40 g (women) to 80 g (men) of ethanol a day for a prolonged period.

Heavy alcohol use affects all organ systems. Apart from the well-known effects on the liver, alcoholism also results in automonic neuropathy, cardiomyopathy, nutritional deficiency, lung injury through aspiration, acute

and chronic pancreatitis and global damage to the central nervous system. Before the onset of impaired hepatic function, alcohol abusers have induced liver microsomal enzymes rendering them resistant to anaesthetic and analgesic agents. (Fig. 2).

Alcohol and surgical morbidity

Alcoholism independently increases the risk of postoperative morbidity 2–3-fold, with related diseases constituting even further risk. The postulated reasons include impaired T cell immunity, decreased levels of circulating fibrinogen and clotting factors and the direct toxicity of alcohol on myocardial cells. Chronic alcohol abuse leads to continued stimulation of the hypopituitary–adrenal axis, creating an enhanced surgical stress response (see Fig. 3). The increased risk of postoperative

morbidity is significantly reduced by one 1 month's preoperative abstinence.

Acute intoxication

It is not unusual for patients to be inebriated when presenting for emergency surgery. There is impaired consciousness and increased sensitivity to hypnotic agents. Full stomach and blunted protective reflexes increase the risk of aspiration. The possibility of other substances of abuse and organ dysfunction from chronic alcoholism should be considered. Hypoglycaemia is a common cause of coma in alcoholics and blood glucose should be monitored regularly and intravenous glucose given if required. Inebriated patients should not receive metronidazole or cephamandole, as they inhibit the enzyme aldehyde dehydrogenase (Fig. 2) leading to increased concentrations of acetaldehyde, a toxic substance.

Alcohol withdrawal

Alcohol withdrawal syndrome is a life threatening medical emergency. The presentation may vary in severity ranging from anxiety, tremor and vomiting to delirium tremens, convulsions, hallucinations and coma. Treatment is with benzodiazepines, fluids, dextrose and nutritional support. Thiamine (100 mg/day) and multivitamins should be given. In an emergency setting withdrawal can be prevented by chlordiazepoxide 10–50 mg p.o. or iv given every 4 hours as needed. The dose can be reduced by 25–50 mg each day.

Cannabis

Cannabis is the most widely used illicit drug in the UK. It induces relaxation and

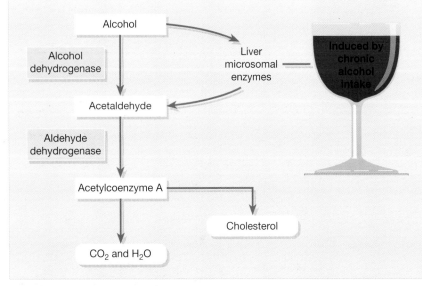

Alcohol

Alcohol dehydrogenase

Acetaldehyde

Aldehyde dehydrogenase

Acetylcoenzyme A

Liver microsomal enzymes

Induced by chronic alcohol intake

Cholesterol

CO_2 and H_2O

Fig. 2 **Alcohol metabolism.**

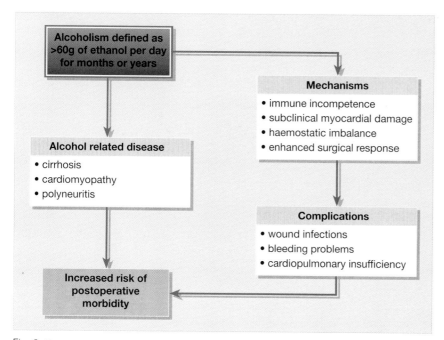

Fig. 3 **Postoperative morbidity and alcoholism.**

contains a number of psychoactive compounds with hallucinogenic effects, including altered perception of sights and sounds. Cannabis is reasonably safe in overdose and withdrawal symptoms are rare. Both the acute and chronic effects on the respiratory system are similar to those of tobacco. The combination of cigarette and marijuana smoking is common and there is additive damage to the lungs. Severe chronic obstructive pulmonary disease may occur.

Postoperative chest infection may require physiotherapy and antibiotics. Care should be exercised in the administration of cerebral depressants and opiates as their effects may be exaggerated by cannabis.

Heroin (diamorphine)

Intravenous drug users present a gamut of challenges to the physician (Fig. 4). They are in a high-risk group for infection with HIV and hepatitis viruses. Repeated needle usage results in venous and arterial thrombosis, the consequences of which may be threatened limbs and systemic infections. Achieving intravenous access is invariably difficult in these patients and expert help may be required. Right-sided infective endocarditis, particularly affecting the tricuspid valve, must always be suspected.

Chronic opiate use results in tolerance, presenting the physician with the dilemma whether the increased opiate demand is related to decreased efficacy or

to desire of the heroin user to satisfy the addiction. Regional analgesia with local anaesthetics is a useful technique in this setting. The acute hospital admission may not be the ideal opportunity to combat addiction, and adequate dosages should be prescribed to alleviate pain and to prevent acute withdrawal. A methadone regime, ranging from 10–60 mg daily, may be instituted as prophylaxis against withdrawal.

Cocaine

Cocaine is a powerful cerebral stimulant, which produces a sense of

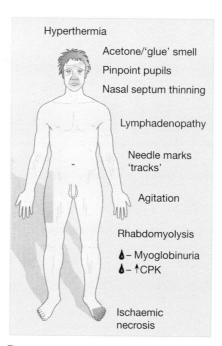

Fig. 4 **Clinical signs of substance misuse.**

euphoria and well-being. Its effects can be fatal, causing cerebral haemorrhage, myocardial infarction and severe hypertension, which can lead to aortic rupture and convulsions.

Drugs such as ephedrine and epinephrine (adrenaline), which lower the threshold for arrhythmias or have sympathomimetic action, should be avoided. In the perioperative period, the cocaine may cause a syndrome, which may be difficult to distinguish from malignant hyperthermia. Like suxemethonium, cocaine is metabolized by pseudo-cholinesterase, and people with a deficiency in this enzyme may have increased susceptibility to cocaine toxicity.

Ecstasy (MDMA)

Ecstasy is popular among young people and produces mild euphoria, relaxation and alteration of perception. It has been associated with fatal hyperthermia, cardiac arrhythmias, renal failure, electrolyte derangement, liver damage and cerebral oedema caused by water intoxication. The presenting features associated with ecstasy abuse may also be confused with malignant hyperthermia.

Clinical case 10

A 46-year-old male with a strong history of alcohol consumption is admitted to the general surgical ward. In the early hours of the morning he becomes confused and agitated. He is irritable, tremulous, sweating profusely and has pulled out his intravenous line. Pulse is 83 beats/min, blood pressure is 110/70 and respiratory rate is 22 breaths/min. How should he be managed?
See comment on page 122-123.

Alcohol and substance abuse

- Alcoholism increases perioperative risk.
- Blood glucose should be checked where there is a history of excessive alcohol use
- Alcohol withdrawal syndrome is a life-threatening emergency.
- Cocaine causes marked increase in sympathetic tone with its attendant problems.
- Water and electrolyte derangement follow ecstasy ingestion.

Oxygen and hypoxia

Human beings cannot survive without oxygen. The brain, in particular, is able to sustain but a brief period of anaerobic (without oxygen) metabolism, after which cellular respiration grinds to a halt and death follows. Unlike other energy substrates, oxygen has a limited storage reserve, with enough oxygen in the blood and the lungs to last only a few minutes. It is therefore imperative that there is an uninterrupted entry of oxygen into the body and a constant delivery of this oxygen to various organ systems. Vulnerability to oxygen deprivation is accentuated during the perioperative period, when the oxygen demand increases and tissue supply may be impaired.

Hypoxia and hypoxaemia

Hypoxia can be defined as insufficient oxygen to meet metabolic needs. Hypoxaemia is decreased partial pressure of oxygen in arterial blood (PaO_2).

Atmospheric oxygen is transported via the lungs, where it crosses into the bloodstream to be taken up by carrier red cell haemoglobin. The heart circulates oxygenated blood to target organs and oxygen diffuses into cell mitochondria, where energy is generated via aerobic (with oxygen) metabolism.

Hypoxic hypoxia

Hypoxic hypoxia occurs in the following situations:

- inadequate inspired oxygen
- hypoventilation
- ventilation–perfusion mismatch (dead space and shunt)
- diffusion abnormality.

Oxygen is present in the air we breathe, usually at a fixed proportion of 21% (FiO_2 ($FiO_2 = 0.21$). Atmospheric pressure is 101 KPa (760 mmHg) at sea level and decreases as altitude increases. Although FiO_2 remains 0.21 at high altitudes, there is a decrease in oxygen partial pressure (Fig. 1).

Hypoventilation occurs commonly following surgery for several reasons. Opiates and anaesthetic agents depress the brainstem ventilatory drive, while pain, weakness or impaired mechanics can prevent efficient breathing. With hypoventilation, there is impaired voiding of CO_2 from the alveoli. The resultant increase in CO_2 partial pressure leads to a decrease in alveolar oxygen. The provision of supplementary oxygen (by increasing the FiO_2) may prevent hypoxaemia (Fig. 2).

Even when breathing is efficient, inspired oxygen may not reach the bloodstream. In the perioperative period, or in some disease processes, areas of the lung may not be ventilated at all. Examples include basal lung collapse, aspiration, pulmonary infarction and alveolar exudates (pulmonary oedema, haemorrhage and pneumonia).

The term shunt refers to the perfusion of unventilated areas. Blood bypassing the lungs completely is termed extrapulmonary shunting. The low arterial oxygen tension with shunting improves only mildly with supplementary oxygen therapy.

Dead space is the ventilation of lung regions without blood flow. In the large airways, this is normal and is termed anatomical dead space, but it is pathological when there is

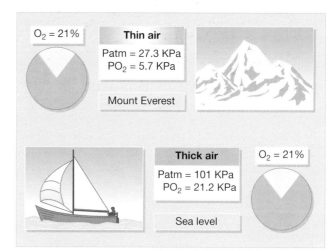

Fig. 1 **Oxygen comprises 21% of air.** As atmospheric pressure decreases, oxygen tension (partial pressure) decreases proportionally.

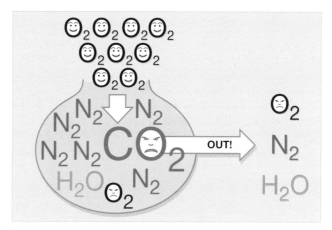

Fig. 2 **The build-up of CO_2 displaces other gases from the alveolus.** Supplementary O_2 increases the proportion and partial pressure of alveolar oxygen, mainly by displacing nitrogen.

inadequate alveolar perfusion. Decreased cardiac output is an example of global dead space, while pulmonary emboli cause local regions of dead space ventilation.

Clinical tip

When patients are given supplementary oxygen, the peripheral oxygen saturation may be normal even in the presence of major lung pathology. This concept is important because there may be a steady worsening of lung function, which is missed until the saturation begins to fall, at which time the patient is in extremis. Arterial blood gases should be checked when in doubt.

Stagnant and anaemic hypoxia

Stagnant hypoxia results from inadequate blood flow. Anaemic hypoxia refers to inadequate carriage of oxygen in the blood. In order for oxygen to arrive at the tissues it must be delivered from the lungs to the tissues. Oxygen delivery is dependent on cardiac output and oxygen content within the

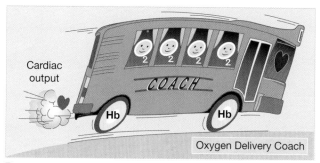

Fig. 3 **Oxygen delivery is dependent on Cardiac Output And Carriage by Haemoglobin.** Otherwise stated, oxygen delivery = cardiac output × oxygen content.

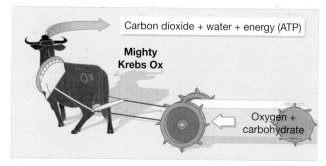

Fig. 5 **Aerobic respiration occurs in the mitochondrion.** Oxygen and fuel (such as glucose) are consumed to power metabolic processes including the Krebs cycle and oxidative phosphorylation. ATP energy is produced and carbon dioxide is a waste product.

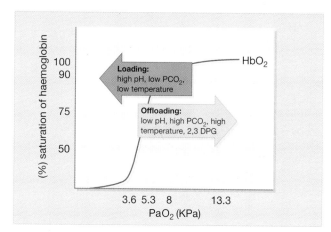

Fig. 4 **Oxyhaemoglobin dissociation curve.**

and all patients should receive supplementary oxygen following major operations. Oxygen therapy may provide the additional benefits of decreasing nausea and vomiting, and decreasing the incidence of wound infections.

Hypoxia should be suspected whenever patients are cyanosed, confused, agitated, unconscious, fitting, not breathing, hypotensive, hypertensive, or there is an arrhythmia, abnormal heart rate or cardiac ischaemia. A pulse oximeter may confirm the diagnosis of hypoxaemia. Lactic acidosis is highly suggestive of tissue hypoxia.

Hypoxia is a medical emergency, which requires urgent treatment with 100% oxygen. Airway support, assisted ventilation and other resuscitative measures may be indicated.

blood (Fig. 3). Apart from impaired oxygen delivery, low cardiac output is also associated with dead space ventilation, as explained above.

Oxygen dissolves poorly in blood, therefore oxygen carriage is dependent on adequate amounts of the efficient carrier molecule, haemoglobin. Impaired oxygen delivery secondary to anaemia is unusual even in sick patients when the haemoglobin concentration exceeds 8 g/dl. Haemoglobin loads O_2 optimally when O_2 tension is high, CO_2 tension is low and pH is high, conditions that are present in pulmonary capillary blood. Offloading of O_2 is facilitated under opposite conditions, as are present in the tissues. This is illustrated graphically in the oxyhaemoglobin dissociation curve (Fig. 4).

Histotoxic hypoxia

When oxygen arrives in the cellular mitochondria, it is used as a substrate for aerobic metabolism (Fig. 5). If the metabolic pathways themselves are dysfunctional, examples being sepsis or cyanide poisoning, then hypoxia results even in the presence of adequate oxygen.

Manifestations and treatment of hypoxia

As there are many tenuous links in the oxygen chain, it is not surprising that hypoxia occurs frequently following surgery,

Hazards of oxygen

The hazards of oxygen therapy are frequently overstated. It is unusual for patients with obstructive airways disease to stop breathing because they are given oxygen. Oxygen toxicity is really only a problem when high concentrations are given over a long period.

Clinical case 11

A young woman has broken her tibia 36 hours ago and is now breathless, confused and cyanosed. She has petechiae in her axillae and on her chest wall. A pulse oximeter shows a saturation of 82%. On a 60% oxygen mask, her saturation increases to 92% and a blood gas shows $PaO_2 = 8.5$ KPa. What is the probable diagnosis?
See comment on page 123.

Oxygen and hypoxia

- Hypoxia is one of the major causes of morbidity and mortality following surgery.

- Hypoxia may be classified according to the cause: hypoxic hypoxia, stagnant hypoxia, anaemic hypoxia and histotoxic hypoxia.

- When supplementary oxygen is given, normal arterial oxygen saturation does not exclude impaired lung function.

- Oxygen therapy is safe, cheap and effective, and should be administered to all patients following major operations.

Acid–base abnormalities

Acid–base abnormalities are frequently observed in the perioperative period. Acid–base abnormalities have either a metabolic or respiratory cause. There are compensatory mechanisms, which attempt to maintain blood pH as close to 7.4 as possible. These include buffers, ventilation, hepatic and renal responses.

Definitions

- Acidaemia is a blood pH < 7.36.
- Alkalaemia is a blood pH > 7.44.
- Acidosis is a process, either metabolic or respiratory, whereby the pH in the blood is decreased.
- Alkalosis is a process whereby the pH in the blood is increased (Fig. 1).

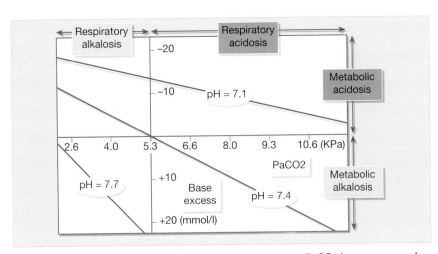

Fig. 1   **Davenport diagram showing the relationships between PaCO$_2$, base excess and blood pH.**

Metabolic acidosis

Metabolic acids include all the body's acids apart from carbon dioxide (CO_2), which forms carbonic acid. Metabolic acidosis often occurs perioperatively. When there is insufficient cellular oxygen (O_2) delivery, cells resort to anaerobic metabolism, which results in lactic acidosis. A useful tool for determining the cause of metabolic acidosis is the 'anion gap' (AG). The AG is the difference between measured cations (sodium and potassium) and anions (chloride and bicarbonate). A normal AG is 12–18 mmol/l.

When there is a metabolic acidosis, bicarbonate is usually decreased. If chloride is unchanged, the anion gap is increased. Causes of high-AG metabolic acidosis include lactic acidosis, ketoacidosis, renal failure, and drugs or toxic substances (such as aspirin, methanol, and ethylene glycol). Normal-AG acidosis occurs when the chloride increase matches the bicarbonate decrease. Hyperchloraemic or normal AG acidosis may result from diarrhoea, renal tubular acidosis, drugs (acetazolamide) and bowel fistulae. Importantly, infusions of normal saline, which has equal amounts of sodium and chloride, potassium chloride or calcium chloride, may result in a hyperchloraemic metabolic acidosis.

Respiratory acidosis

Respiratory acidosis is present when PaCO$_2$ (carbon dioxide tension in arterial blood) is elevated (Fig. 2). The lungs eliminate about 16 000 mmol of carbonic acid as CO_2 daily, while the kidneys dispose of only 100 mmol of acid a day. Thus, derangement and compensation can occur much more rapidly via ventilatory than via renal routes.

Opiates are potent centrally acting ventilatory depressants and are frequently the cause of respiratory acidosis perioperatively. Residual effects of muscle relaxants after surgery also prevent efficient ventilation causing respiratory acidosis.

Problems resulting from acidaemia

Severe acidaemia may cause confusion, coma, impaired cardiac contractility, cardiac arrhythmia, reduced threshold for ventricular fibrillation, decreased

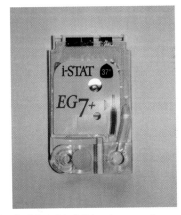

Fig. 2   **A hand-held blood gas analyser cartridge.** Heparinized syringes are used to prevent clotting of blood in the machine.

hepatic and renal blood flow, hyperkalaemia (see Fig. 3) and right shift of the oxyhaemoglobin dissociation curve. Respiratory acidosis also leads to increased cerebral blood flow and raised intracranial pressure. In severe acidaemia (pH < 7.2), the heart and the vasculature are less responsive to catecholamines.

Treatment of acidaemia

The priority is to identify and treat the underlying cause. Oxygen, fluid resuscitation and blood may all be required. In ketoacidosis and lactic acidosis treating the underlying disorder may result in conversion of the accumulated anions to bicarbonate. By contrast in hyperchloraemic acidosis (normal AG), there is usually a loss of bicarbonate (e.g. diarrhoea). These patients benefit from alkali therapy with sodium bicarbonate. The formula for calculating dosage is 0.3 × body mass

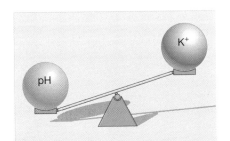

Fig. 3   **Diagram showing the relationship between pH and plasma potassium.**

(Kg) × base deficit. (negative base excess). Bicarbonate is only indicated in life-threatening acidosis. Acidaemia may also be treated with haemodialysis.

Problems with bicarbonate

- The majority is converted to CO_2. Thus adequate cardiac output and normal ventilation are required.
- CO_2 may freely enter cells and worsen intracellular acidosis.
- Alkalosis, hypernatraemia, and hyperosmolality may result.

Metabolic alkalosis

A loss of acid (hydrogen ions) or a gain in bicarbonate cause metabolic alkalosis. Hydrogen may be lost from gastric fluid or in the urine. Patients on thiazide or loop diuretics, or those who have been vomiting, frequently develop a metabolic alkalosis. Bicarbonate gain may result from inappropriate and overzealous treatment of acidosis, and may also occur in sepsis.

Respiratory alkalosis

Respiratory alkalosis is the most frequently encountered acid–base disorder, since it occurs in normal pregnancy and at high altitudes. In disease it occurs as a reflex attempt to compensate for primary metabolic acidosis or for hypoxaemia. Salicylate intoxication, hepatic failure, sepsis, and the anxiety-hyperventilation–syndrome are additional causes of respiratory alkalosis.

Problems resulting from alkalaemia

Alkalaemia may lead to impaired cerebral perfusion, headache, tetany, seizures, delirium, stupor, coma and death. The associated reduction in the plasma concentration of ionized calcium contributes to some of these manifestations. Metabolic alkalosis depresses ventilation, causing hypercapnia and hypoxaemia.

Hypokalaemia is an almost constant feature of alkalaemic disorders, but it is more prominent in those of metabolic origin. Hypokalaemia can have several adverse effects, including neuromuscular weakness, arrhythmias, polyuria, and increased ammonia production. Acute alkalaemia can reduce

the release of oxygen to the tissues by tightening the binding of oxygen to haemoglobin.

Treatment of metabolic alkalosis

Most severe metabolic alkalosis is of the chloride-responsive form, the most common causes being loss of gastric acid and the administration of loop or thiazide diuretics. If the processes that generate metabolic alkalosis are ongoing, every effort should be made to moderate or stop them. Vomiting should be countered with antiemetics. If continuation of gastric drainage is required, administering H_2-receptor blockers or inhibitors of the gastric proton pump can reduce the loss of gastric acid. Decreasing the dose of loop

or thiazide diuretics should be coupled with the addition of a potassium-sparing diuretic. Patients with volume depletion require provision of both sodium chloride and potassium chloride. Haemodialysis and ultrafiltration can rapidly correct severe alkalaemia.

Drugs and acid–base abnormalities

Variation in pH alters the ionization of proteins and drugs. Generally, ionized drugs cannot readily cross cell membranes. For example, an acidic environment caused by local sepsis impairs the action of local anaesthetics. In contrast, alkalaemia potentiates the action of morphine and pethidine by increasing un-ionized fractions of these drugs (Fig. 4).

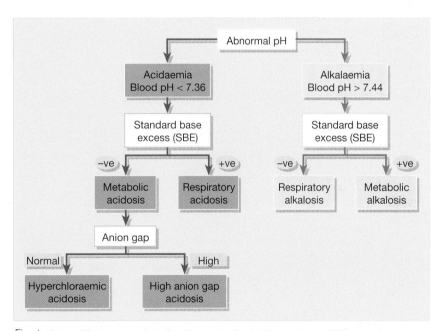

Fig. 4 **A simplified approach to the diagnosis of acid–base abnormalities.**

Clinical case 12

A 60-year-old man presents for elective orthopaedic surgery. He has been taking frusemide for hypertension for 3 years. His arterial blood gas reveals: pH = 7.505, PCO_2 = 6.5 KPa, PO_2 = 11.31 KPa, HCO_3a = 32.6 mmol/l, HCO_3S = 30.5 mmol/l, BE = 6.6 mmol/l, Na = 133 mmol/l, K = 3.01 mmol/l, Cl = 94 mmol/l. Interpret the blood gas and suggest how the abnormalities may be treated.
See comment on page 123.

Acid–base abnormalities

- The terms acidaemia and alkalaemia refer to abnormalities in blood pH, whereas acidosis and alkalosis refer to processes by which pH is altered.
- Both metabolic and respiratory acidosis occur frequently following surgery.
- The diagnosis of acid–base disturbance is based on arterial blood gas analysis coupled with clinical history and examination.
- The priority is to treat the underlying cause of the disturbance.
- Chemical treatment or haemodialysis to correct acidaemia or alkalaemia is indicated only when patients are critically ill.

Carbon dioxide

Abnormal arterial blood carbon dioxide ($PaCO_2$) following surgery has important consequences for the functioning of various organ systems. Carbon dioxide (CO_2) is produced during cellular respiration and must be transported to the lungs where it can be blown off. CO_2 is carried in blood in three forms: dissolved, bound to proteins, and as bicarbonate (HCO_3). When haemoglobin offloads oxygen (O_2) to the tissues, the ability of blood to carry CO_2 improves, which is termed the Haldane effect. Oxygenation of blood in the lungs facilitates the elimination of CO_2. Through homeostatic regulation, PaCO2 is maintained roughly between 5–5.5 KPa (37–41 mmHg). The major stimuli for increasing ventilation are acidaemia, low oxygen tension (PO_2), and elevated PCO_2, with PCO_2 being the most potent stimulus.

Alveolar ventilation is under the control of ventilatory centres in the pons and medulla oblongata (Fig. 1). Changes in the production of CO_2 are accompanied by corresponding alterations in alveolar ventilation, resulting in little or no change in $PaCO_2$. Ventilation is regulated by brainstem chemoreceptors for PCO_2, PO_2, and pH, by neural impulses from arterial chemoreceptors and lung-stretch receptors and by impulses from the cerebral cortex.

Hypercapnia

Hypercapnia (elevated $PaCO_2$) may occur when CO_2 production increases, transport to the lung is impaired, or ventilation is inefficient. In hypermetabolic states, there is a steep increase in CO_2 generation. Examples include sepsis, burns, exercise, fever, hyperthyroidism, malignant hyperthermia, and phaeochromocytoma. When cardiac output is reduced, CO_2 delivery to the lungs is impaired.

Pulmonary emboli, in addition to placing a strain on the heart, block vessels and prevent blood flow to ventilated regions.

Several factors may result in hypoventilation, (see Fig. 1), some of which are especially pertinent in the perioperative period. Diaphragmatic weakness and splinting occurs following abdominal surgery. Anaesthetic agents, opiates and sedatives decrease the sensitivity of the ventilatory centre to CO_2. Other causes of hypercapnia include airway obstruction, brainstem injury, neuromuscular weakness, pulmonary disease and circulatory impairment.

Central nervous system

Hypercapnia causes profound generalized vasodilatation. There is resulting increased cerebral blood flow with concomitant rise in cerebral blood volume. Compliance of the cranium is poor and, when there is elevated intracranial pressure (ICP), the increase in blood volume may have devastating consequences. As CO_2 increases, patients may become agitated, confused and eventually somnolent (see Fig. 2). At very high levels CO_2 can actually cause narcosis. There is a lowering of the seizure threshold and hypercapnia may cause fitting.

Cardiovascular and pulmonary systems

Hypercapnia induces catecholamine release and stimulation of the sympathetic nervous system resulting in tachycardia, myocardial ischaemia and cardiac arrhythmias. Cardiac output increases with generalized vasodilatation, but severe respiratory acidosis compromises myocardial contractility. Interestingly, there is evidence suggesting that mild hypercapnia may protect the heart against ischaemic injury. Because hypercapnia increases cardiac output, oxygen delivery is increased throughout the body.

Pulmonary system

Pulmonary vasoconstriction and pulmonary hypertension are consequences of hypercapnia. Elevated $PaCO_2$ is dangerous for patients with intracardiac shunts as the elevated pulmonary pressure may reverse shunt flow, causing severe hypoxaemia. Marked increase in alveolar CO_2 partial pressure decreases the tension of other alveolar gases, particularly oxygen.

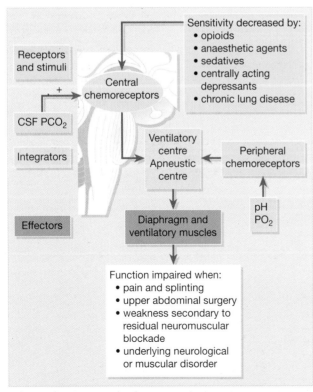

Fig. 1 **Control of ventilation.**

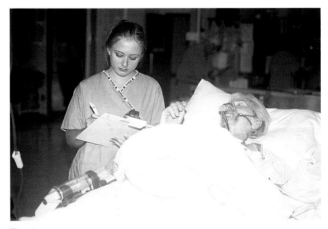

Fig. 2 **Nurse monitoring adequacy of ventilation following surgery.** Parameters assessed include level of consciousness, pain score, rate of breathing, oxygen saturation, blood pressure, heart rate and cardiac rhythm.

Nonetheless, the improved cardiac output coupled with vasoconstriction in poorly oxygenated areas of the lungs may actually improve PaO_2.

Haematological, metabolic and renal effects

Increased $PaCO_2$ shifts the oxyhaemoglobin dissociation curve to the right thereby facilitating the offloading of oxygen, which is termed the Bohr effect.

Retention of bicarbonate by the kidneys is stimulated to compensate for the respiratory acidosis.

Permissive hypercapnia

Mild $PaCO_2$ elevation is well tolerated and results in minimal physiological embarrassment. There is increasing evidence that respiratory (and metabolic) acidosis can exert protective effects on tissue injury, and furthermore, that hypocapnia may be deleterious. High opiate dosage may be required to provide adequate postoperative analgesia. The biggest danger with resulting hypoventilation is hypoxaemia. This can be prevented by the provision of supplementary oxygen. The graphical depiction of the CO_2 response indicates that with sedatives and opiates, the responsiveness is blunted, but there is still adequate ventilation at a higher $PaCO_2$ set point (see Fig. 3).

Hypocapnia

Hyperventilation is the usual cause of hypocapnia. The chief stimuli to hyperventilation are metabolic acidosis and chronic hypoxaemia, as occurs at high altitudes. Iatrogenic hypocapnia is also common. Patients who are on intensive care units or under anaesthesia may receive assisted ventilation with a mechanical ventilator. Intentional hyperventilation is occasionally employed, and accidental hyperventilation frequently occurs.

The causes of acute hypocapnia include hypoxia, anxiety, pain, sepsis, hepatic failure, CNS disorders (such as stroke and infections), pulmonary disorders (including infections and interstitial lung disease), drugs (like salicylate intoxication), and pregnancy.

Acute reduction in PCO_2 produces a small but immediate decrease in bicarbonate due to cellular uptake of bicarbonate in exchange for chloride. Acute hypocapnia also induces cellular uptake of potassium and phosphate, and increases the binding of ionised calcium to serum albumin. Patients with acute hypocapnia may experience cardiac arrhythmias, cerebral vasoconstriction, facial and peripheral paraesthesias, muscle cramps, tetany and syncope or seizures.

Central nervous system

Hypocapnia causes cerebral vasocontriction, leading to decreased cerebral blood flow and blood volume. Acutely, there may be a significant reduction in ICP.

Profound hyperventilation leads to impairment of cerebral perfusion and oxygenation. Even mild hyperventilation may be hazardous in patients with partial stenosis of blood vessels to the brain. There is long-term neurological damage following prolonged dwelling at high altitude, which is probably not a consequence of chronic hypoxaemia, but rather secondary to the generation of extremely low $PaCO_2$.

Cardiovascular and pulmonary systems

Acute respiratory alkalosis may jeopardize coronary perfusion. Generalized vasoconstriction increases afterload and places a strain on the myocardium.

Pulmonary vascular resistance is decreased by hypocapnia, which may be exploited in patients with pulmonary hypertension or cyanotic congenital heart disease. Hypocapnia, however, also increases microvascular permeability in tracheal mucosa, decreases lung compliance, and increases dysfunctional surfactant production. Pulmonary vasodilatation may inappropriately increase blood flow to poorly ventilated lung regions.

Haematological metabolic and renal effects

Hypocapnia shifts the oxyhaemoglobin dissociation curve leftwards, restricting oxygen offloading at the tissue level; local oxygen delivery may be further impaired by hypocapnia-induced vasoconstriction.

There is a respiratory alkalosis and compensatory renal excretion of bicarbonate is encouraged.

Clinical case 13

A 55-year-old man has had upper abdominal surgery. He is receiving morphine for analgesia. The nursing staff, concerned that he is somnolent and not breathing, suggest that naloxone should be administered. He is rouseable and breathing at a rate of six breaths per minute. A blood gas on room air reveals pH = 7.25, $PaCO_2$ = 7.2 KPa (54 mmHg) and PaO_2 = 8.5 Kpa (64 mmHg). There is no haemodynamic compromise and he is otherwise well. Is naloxone the appropriate intervention?
See comment on page 123.

Carbon dioxide

- Carbon dioxide abnormalities develop rapidly and have important physiological consequences.

- The major stimulus for breathing is carbon dioxide.

- Mild hypercapnia is well tolerated and may even have therapeutic applications.

- Supplementary oxygen should be administered to patients who develop acute hypercapnia.

- The body does not adapt well to hypocapnia, which, through profound vasoconstriction, decreases perfusion to vital organs.

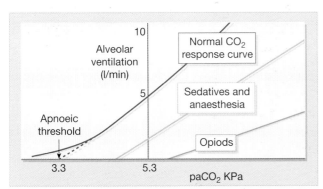

Fig. 3 **CO_2 response curve.** Alveolar ventilation $= K \times PaCO_2 \times CO_2$ production. Alveolar ventilation is directly proportional to $PaCO_2$.

Electrolytes

Electrolyte disorders are potentially life-threatening perioperative complications, sodium and potassium abnormalities being particularly common.

Sodium

Sodium is the most abundant plasma electrolyte. The intracellular store is low, which increases susceptibilty to acute fluctuations in plasma sodium concentration.

The main mechanisms underlying the development of low sodium are loss of sodium from the body (urinary and drain losses) and plasma dilution (water overload). Postoperative hyponatraemia may develop even when isotonic saline is used due to the dilutional effect of anti diuretic hormone (ADH), which is released as part of the stress response to surgery. It is imperative to ensure that patients receive their sodium requirements and those who have even mild hyponatraemia may benefit from hypertonic fluids. Diuretics cause natriuresis, and should be avoided if possible.

Normal saline contains 154 mmol/l of sodium, which is slightly higher than the normal plasma concentration of 135–145 mmol/l. The sodium concentration of normal saline is 0.9% equating to 0.9 g of sodium per 100 ml. A typical hypertonic saline solution has a sodium concentration of 3%. Patients with symptomatic hyponatraemia (Table 1) may benefit from hypertonic saline or water restriction depending upon the severity of the hyponatraemia. Symptoms are more severe if hyponatraemia has developed rapidly.

The aim of treatment should be to raise plasma sodium by no more than 1 mmol/l per hour until symptoms resolve, with a caveat being not to increase the sodium concentration by more than 8 mmol/l/day. This may be achieved by administering 0.5 ml/kg of 3% hypertonic saline hourly. During correction, plasma sodium concentrations should be monitored 2-hourly. Overzealous sodium replacement is exteremely hazardous and may result in central pontine myelinolysis.

Although rare, hypernatraemia (elevated plasma sodium) may also be encountered. The most common cause is the loss of low sodium-containing fluid from the renal or gastrointestinal systems without adequate fluid replacement.

The appropriate treatment of hypernatraemia depends on volume status. In the hypovolaemic patient, the priority is restoration of intravascular volume and haemodynamic stability. Any resuscitation fluid may be used to accomplish this. Once this is achieved, a hypotonic fluid like 5% dextrose may be administered at a rate of 1 l every 6 hours until the hypernatraemia resolves. If there is hypervolaemia, diuretic therapy combined with 5% dextrose as maintenance fluid usually corrects the problem. Oral fluids may be as effective as and safer than intravenous fluids. Care should be taken not to cause hyponatraemia.

Potassium

Potassium is far more abundant inside cells than in plasma. Hypokalaemia is defined as a plasma potassium concentration less than 3.5 mmol/l. Hypokalaemia may result from a variety of causes including diuretic therapy, inadequate dietary potassium, gastrointestinal loss, administration of intravenous fluids that do not contain potassium, and potassium shifts into cells, as occurs with alkalaemia.

Hypokalaemia is hazardous. For those who have cardiovascular disease and those on digoxin therapy, even mild hypokalaemia may precipitate life-threatening cardiac arrhythmias. For patients who are already receiving diuretic therapy the addition of potassium-sparing diuretics may be beneficial. The intake of foods rich in potassium, such as fruit, vegetables and nuts (Fig. 1), may prevent hypokalaemia. If a patient is found to have hypokalaemia during an operation, potassium may be safely administered while the patient is anaesthetized and closely monitored.

Low plasma potassium is usually only the tip of the iceberg, and there is a significant total body potassium deficit. Potassium should always be given as a slow infusion and should not be replaced at a rate exceeding 20–40 mmol/hr in an adult. A rapid intravenous bolus of potassium invariably causes ventricular fibrillation or asystole.

Severe hyerkalaemia may occur with such conditions as renal failure, acidaemia and muscle breakdown. Electocardiogram changes herald imminent malignant cardiac arrhthymias or asystole. The emergency treatment of hyperkalaemia involves administration of calcium to stabilize the myocardial membrane, insulin (with dextrose) to drive potassium into cells and bicarbonate to encourage the intracellular shift of potassium in exchange for hydrogen ions (see Fig. 2 and Fig. 3).

Hypomagnesaemia

Hypomagnesaemia is associated with other electrolyte derangements, especially hypokalaemia and hypocalcaemia. Roughly 65% of patients on intensive care units and 12% of patients on general wards have hypomagnasaemia. Diabetics, alcoholics and those receiving diuretic therapy are at particularly high risk. Magnesium correction may be a prerequisite for the successful treatment of other electrolyte abnormalities. (see Fig. 4)

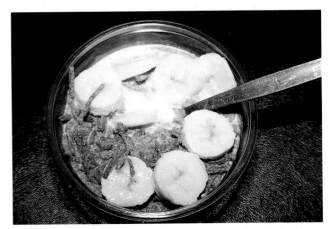

Fig. 1 **The intake of foods rich in potassium may prevent hypokalaemia.**

Table 1 **Manifestations of hyponatraemia**	
Sodium concentration	**Manifestations**
125–160 mmol/l	Usually asymptomatic
115–125 mmol/l	Headache, nausea, vomiting, muscle cramps, lethargy, disorientation, depressed reflexes
< 115 mmol/l	Seizures, coma, brain damage, respiratory arrest, brain stem herniation, death

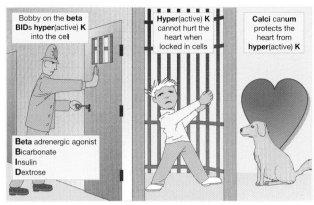

Fig. 2 **Hyperactive K is pushed into the cell by the beta BIDs (beta adrenergic agonist, bicarbonate, insulin and dextrose), and calcium protects the heart from it.**

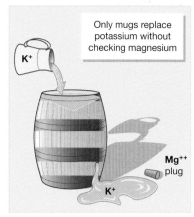

Fig. 4 **Magnesium correction may be a requisite for successful treatment of other electrolyte abnormalities.**

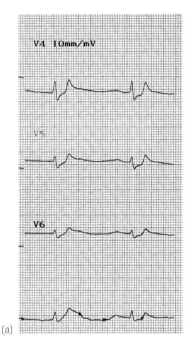

(a)

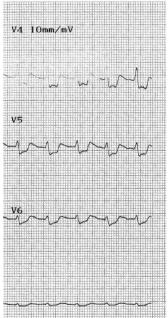

(b)

Calcium

Calcium may be measured as total calcium, corrected calcium (to albumin) and as ionized calcium. Bone is the chief calcium reservoir and hypercalcaemia may occur when calcium is liberated. There are many potential causes including malignancy, immobilization, hyperparathyroidism, sarcoidosis, dehydration, and rhabdomyolysis.

To prevent perioperative hypercalcaemia, generous oral salt and water intake should be encouraged to maintain extracellular volume and to facilitate urinary calcium excretion. Hypercalcaemia has dangerous neurological, gastrointestinal and renal consequences. Loop diuretics may be used to encourage calcium clearance, along with a saline volume loading, thereby returning calcium to the normal range. Depending on the cause of hypercalcaemia other therapies such as steroids, permidronate or dialysis may be indicated.

Low plasma calcium may be caused by shock, trauma, pancreatitis, massive blood transfusion, thyroid and parathyroid surgery and vitamin D deficiency. Complications include hypotension, tetany, QT interval lengthening on the electrocardiogram, heart block and ventricular fibrillation. If a patient does develop symptomatic hypocalcaemia, intravenous calcium is required until signs and symptoms abate.

Fig. 3 **(a) Section of an ECG trace from a patient with hyperkalaemia.** Note the broad QRS complexes and the peaked T waves. With hypokalaemia, the QRS complexes are broad, but the T waves are flat and prominent U waves appear. **(b) The plasma potassium has decreased and the ECG trace has improved following treatment with 10ml 10% calcium gluconate, 50ml 8.4% bicarbonate, 10 units of insulin and 50 ml 50% glucose.**

Clinical case 14

A 64-year-old woman with mild hypertension has been on diuretic therapy and has had a hip replacement 2 days ago. She appears confused and has recently had a seizure. She was vomiting following the operation and has been given 4 l of 5% dextrose solution in order to maintain the intravascular volume. She is haemodynamically stable and the haemoglobin is 9 g/dl. What is the most likely diagnosis and how should she be treated?
See comment on page 123.

Electrolytes

■ Electrolytes should be within the normal ranges before elective surgery.

■ Underlying causes of the abnormalities should be addressed.

■ Electrolyte abnormalities may be refractory to correction if other abnormalities are not simultaneously treated.

■ Complications of rapid correction may be more devastating than the complications of the initial derangement.

Temperature

The temperature of the major organs of the body is maintained within narrow limits ($\pm 0.2°C$) around a set-point of $37°C$. This set-point has diurnal variations from $36.5°C$ in the morning to $37.5°C$ in the evening. When core temperature is at the set-point thermoregulatory reflexes are least active. In disease, the set-point may be moved up by microbial toxins or other factors, causing a fever. Paracetamol acts by inhibiting local synthesis of prostaglandin, a mediator in the posterior hypothalamus essential for generation of fever. A sudden increase in body temperature acts as a signal broadcast to the whole body, enhancing the immune response.

Regulation of body temperature is achieved mainly through behaviour, i.e. wearing appropriate clothes. The autonomic mechanisms for heat conservation are vasoconstriction and shivering and for heat loss are vasodilatation and sweating. Temperature regulation is masterminded by the hypothalamus receiving inputs from the skin and other parts of the CNS (Fig. 1). The neurotransmitters noradrenaline, 5-hydroxytryptamine, acetylcholine and prostaglandins E1 and E2, all play a part in temperature regulation.

Physical means for exchanging heat with the environment:

- Convection of air.
- Evaporation of sweat see (Fig. 2).
- Radiation and conduction.

There is a balance between the heat produced within the body by metabolism and that lost to the environment through the skin. A mismatch between these two leads either to hypothermia or to hyperthermia.

The definition of body temperature is not straightforward. There is a body core comprising the major organs (brain, heart, etc) tightly regulated around the set-point. Limb muscles may vary their temperature by as much as $4°C$ away from the core. When taking a clinical measurement of temperature the purpose and the site of the measurement must be specified.

Devices for measuring temperature

- *The clinical thermometer* – uses expansion of a liquid (mercury or alcohol)in a tube. Accuracy: $0.1°C$; slow response.
- *Liquid crystal thermometer* – disposable; less accurate than the mercury thermometer but faster electrical devices.
- *Thermistors or thermocouples* – require a box of electronics with a display. Very accurate and fast response allowing a continuous record. Essential for thermodilution methods of blood flow measurement.
- *Remote sensing devices* – sense infrared radiation. Used clinically to measure tympanic temperature by a hand-held device. Infrared cameras in clinical thermography shows 'hot' and 'cold' areas on the surface of the body.

Failure of temperature regulation

Severe hyperthermia or hypothermia are usually managed in the ICU. Core temperatures $> 42°C$ are fatal. Below $30°C$ there is a high chance of ventricular fibrillation. Hypothermia and hyperthermia may be deliberately induced for therapeutic purposes.

Effects of hypothermia ($< 34°C$) on the body include:

- Decreased immunity
- Decreased muscle power and metabolic rate
- Increased N_2 loss
- Decreased blood clotting
- Decreased threshold of pain
- Increased duration of effect of drugs
- Protection from effects of ischaemia
- Ventricular fibrillation ($< 31°C$)
- Acid–base disturbances.

Effects of hyperthermia include:

- Increased metabolic rate, O_2 consumption and CO_2 production
- Increased cardiac work
- Increased fluid requirement
- Increased CNS excitability (seizures in children).

Hypothermia

Hypothermia is usually accidental, due to exposure. Old people and small children are most susceptible. Treatment is conservative, allowing natural mechanisms to restore body temperature slowly. In severe cases, disturbances in plasma electrolytes and

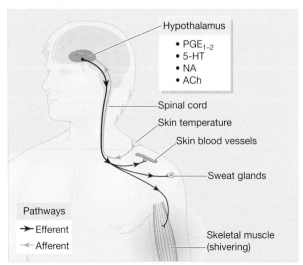

Fig. 1 **The anterior hypothalamus is concerned with heat loss and the posterior with heat conservation.** Specific thermal receptors (warm and cold) are in the skin, spinal cord, and hypothalamus.

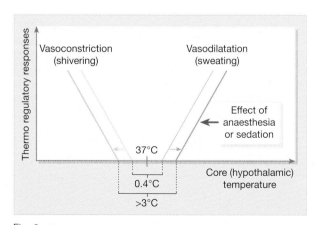

Fig. 2 **Diagram representing the intensity of thermoregulatory responses in a normal patient.** No responses are detectable as long as core temperature remains at $37\pm0.2°C$. Anaesthesia or sedation 'blunt' the responses in a dose-dependent manner. During surgical anaesthesia there may be no responses in the range $34–40°C$.

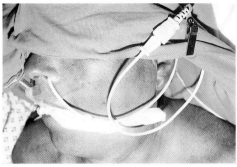
(a)

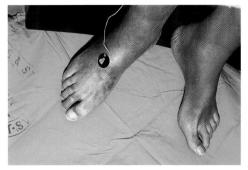
(b)

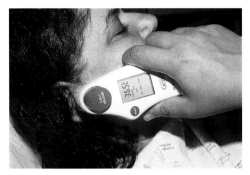
(c)

Fig. 3 **Thermometres. (a)** Clinical thermometer. **(b)** Electric sensor. **(c)** Tympanic sensor.

in acid–base balance should be corrected.

General anaesthetics (e.g. propofol) and opioids (e.g. fentanyl) depress the hypothalamic threshold for peripheral vasoconstriction and shivering by 2–3°C and neuromuscular blockers abolish heat production in muscle. There is a rapid redistribution of heat from the core to the periphery during the first 30 minutes of general anaesthesia causing a 1–2°C decrease in core temperature. An equilibrium is reached when the heat loss to the environment is balanced by internal heat production.

There are no means to prevent the initial redistributive decrease in core temperature other than keeping the patient in a warm environment just before anaesthesia. On awakening from anaesthesia, the effects of drugs wear off while the core is still hypothermic causing reflex vasoconstriction and shivering, often seen postoperatively.

There is an increase in oxygen requirement during shivering, which may be dangerous. Administration of oxygen and application of whole-body warming devices are helpful.

Hyperthermia

Hyperthermia may be caused by excessive heat production, decreased heat dissipation, or malfunction of the hypothalamic thermostat. Usually it is caused by infection and is known as *fever or pyrexia*. Fever in excess of 39°C is an indication for antipyretic therapy in patients with underlying diseases. Paracetamol or aspirin are the agents of choice, except in small children with influenza or varicella, where aspirin should be avoided because it may precipitate Reye's syndrome. Ibuprofen is an alternative.

In the setting of anaesthesia or ICU, hyperthermia may be caused by accidental overheating due to breakdown of control of heating devices or by a rare complication known as 'malignant hyperthermia'. This is a form of familial autosomal-dominant myopathy which may be triggered by volatile anaesthetics or by suxamethonium (a neuromuscular blocker). A family history is the most important clue to susceptibility and a muscle biopsy for contracture test is the best way to screen for susceptibility. The syndrome is often fatal, even when diagnosed. The pathophysiology includes a loss of control of the permeability to Ca^{2+} in the sarcoplasmic reticulum in skeletal muscle, leading to a contracture and an exaggerated metabolic demand. Supportive measures and dantrolene are the mainstay of management.

Exertional hyperthermia

Exertional hyperthermia is a response to intense exercise. In marathon runners rectal temperatures of 39–40°C are common. Heat-stroke occurs in sedentary, elderly persons or the very young. Predisposing factors include obesity, the use of anticholinergics or diuretics and dehydration during a heat-wave. The clinical features of heat-stroke include an acute onset, core temperature above 40°C, delirium, stupor or coma, hypotension, tachycardia, and hyperventilation. There is hemoconcentration, proteinuria and microscopical haematuria, and abnormal liver function. Muscle-enzyme levels are elevated. Respiratory alkalosis and hypokalemia occur early and lactic acidosis and hyperkalemia occur later. The mortality rate for heat-stroke is high. Management includes the application of cool water to the body surface, and oral or intravenous hydration.

Neuroleptic malignant syndrome

The neuroleptic malignant syndrome occurs in about 0.2% of patients who receive neuroleptic agents, usually within the first 30 days of therapy. Haloperidol is the most common cause, but widely used anti-emetics such as metoclopramide may be responsible The syndrome is triggered by the blockade of dopaminergic receptors in the corpus striatum, resulting in spasticity of the skeletal muscle and impaired hypothalamic-mediated heat dissipation. Treatment is supportive and requires withdrawal of the causing agent. The mortality rate is about 20%. A similar syndrome may be triggered by self-poisoning with 'ecstasy' (MDMA). Hyperthermia and muscle rigidity are the usual presenting symptoms and if core temperature reaches > 40°C the syndrome is often fatal. It occurs unpredictably and is not dose-related.

Clinical case 15

In the surgical ward a 72-year-old male patient is complaining of pain and is found shivering 90 minutes after a transurethral resection of the prostate gland.
See comment on page 123.

Temperature

- Hypothermia – is usually accidental, common during and after surgery, protective against the effects of ischaemia, may cause ventricular fibrillation and is best treated by removing the cause and supportive measures.

- Hyperthermia – usually results from infection (fever), may be accidental (heat-stroke), may be drug-induced (high mortality) and includes malignant hyperpyrexia and neuroleptic malignant syndrome.
  - Fever > 39°C treated with paracetamol.
  - Drug-induced: dantrolene and physical cooling.

The elderly

Improvements in social conditions and in healthcare mean that people live longer. In England and Wales in 1900 4% of the population was aged 65 or over. In 1990 that proportion had risen to 16% and by 2020 that figure will rise to 20%. An increasing proportion of healthcare resource will have to be directed towards the elderly. Healthcare workers need to have a thorough understanding of the medical, physiological and psychological changes brought about by ageing.

There are changes in the anatomy and in the physiology of the body associated with ageing which are initiated by genetic determinants and accelerated by environmental factors. Such environmental factors include smoking, poor diet, alcohol, sunlight and ionizing radiation.

Special perioperative considerations

Important systems affected by ageing include (see Fig. 1):

Autonomic nervous system
- There is an increased risk of perioperative hypothermia, because of less efficient temperature control.
- Ventilatory responses to hypoxia and hypercarbia are impaired and are further blunted by narcotic and sedative drugs. There is increased risk both of carbon dioxide retention and of hypoxia, both of which may contribute to POCD (see below).
- The reflexes that control blood pressure become blunted with ageing, failing to maintain blood pressure in response to acute haemorrhage or fluid loss.

Cardiovascular and respiratory systems
- Cardiovascular ageing includes 'hardening of the arteries' and a decrease in myocardial ability to increase work,

impairing the responses to raised metabolic demands, to haemorrhage or acute fluid loss.
- Respiratory ageing reduces not only the efficiency of gas exchange and the mechanical ability to move air in and out of the lungs, but also the ability to increase ventilation in response to raised metabolic demand. Laryngeal reflexes that protect the bronchial tree and lungs from ingress of fluid, food and vomit are also impaired. Sedation increases the risk of aspiration pneumonia.

Kidneys and renal function
- There is a loss in numbers of nephrons and disruption of renal tubules. This results in an impaired ability to excrete water-soluble waste products and drug metabolites, to handle fluid overload and to secrete acid.
- The kidneys become more susceptible to injury following hypotension or dehydration.

Co-existent disease
Age increases the likelihood of other diseases occurring in parallel with the condition requiring surgery. The commonest conditions are cardiovascular or respiratory. Ischaemic heart disease, hypertension and chronic obstructive pulmonary disease are common. The conditions listed in Table 1 can alter an individual's response to surgery and anaesthesia, while drugs used to treat some of these conditions can interact with anaesthetic agents.

Table 1 Conditions which may alter an elderly patient's response to surgery and anaesthesia	
Common ailments of old age	**Common treatment**
Hypertension	Anti-hypertensives
Heart Failure	Diuretics
Atrial fibrillation	Digoxin
Chronic obstructive pulmonary disease	Bronchodilators
Non-insulin dependent diabetes	Oral hypoglycaemics
Hypothyroidism	Thyroxine
Agitation, depression	Antidepressants, sedatives

Drug handling and drug dosages
Ageing may affect drug action and drug elimination in two ways:

- *Compartment changes* – there is a reduction in body water and an increase in the proportion of body fat. Many drugs administered in a dose calculated on a mg/kg basis will achieve a higher concentration at their site of action due to the reduction in body water, and so appear to have an increased potency. The increase in the proportion of body fat enhances drug sequestration, so slowing elimination.
- *Hepatic biotransformation* of drugs and renal elimination of water-soluble products become less efficient, resulting in prolonged clearance time, e.g. diazepam.

The overall effect of these changes is to increase apparent drug potency and prolong duration of drug action (see Table 2).

Bones, joints and posture
Progressive loss of protein matrix and de-mineralization results in a reduction of bone strength and increased chance of fractures. Osteoarthritis is common and the normal thoracic kyphosis may become exaggerated necessitating use of pillows to support the head when lying supine.

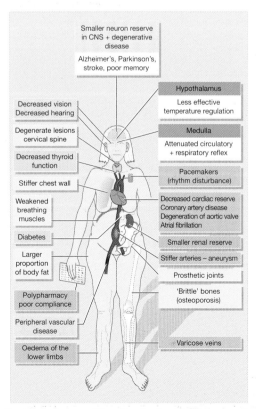

Fig. 1 **Perioperative considerations in the elderly.**

Table 2 **Issues relevant to the elderly during the conduct of anaesthesia**	
Factor	Action
Drug dose	Reduce dose and frequency
Fluids	Avoid fluid overload
Limbs	Care with positioning, protect bony prominences
Posture	Care with joints that are stiff or limited in movement
Heat loss	Reduce heat loss, employ active warming
Venous access	Use non-dominant limb, beware vessel fragility

Table 3 **Abbreviated mental test (AMT)**
1. Age
2. Time (to nearest hour)
3. Address for recall at end of test (e.g. 41 East Street). Patient should be asked to repeat address immediately to ensure that it was heard correctly.
4. Year
5. Name of hospital
6. Recognition of two people (e.g. nurse, doctor)
7. Date of birth
8. Year of start of World War 1 (or equivalent national event)
9. Name of Monarch/Head of State
10. Count backwards from 20 to 1

Social factors

Age related psychosocial changes may result in social isolation, behavioural idiosyncrasies, agitation and fear or suspicion of strangers, including medical and nursing attendants. Colloquial expressions used by younger generations may be the cause of misunderstandings, particularly when associated with hearing problems and/or impaired short-term memory. There may be an unwillingness to complain about pain or other symptoms (stoicism) so that postoperative pain may be left untreated.

Preoperative assessment

The following provide useful information:

- Co-existent medical problems.
- Basic cognitive assessment.
- Current medication.
- Cardiovascular and respiratory status.
- Haemoglobin and electrolyte results.
- Chest X-Ray and ECG.
- Abbreviated Mental Test (AMT) (Table 3).

Obtaining a thorough medical history may be difficult for several reasons. These include deafness, memory loss, anxiety, confusion, cognitive disorder, language barrier, cultural difference and poor dentition. Patience and courtesy are of paramount importance. A simple test of cognitive function (AMT) can be performed pre- and postoperatively. A preoperative score below 7 may indicate pre-existing dementia, while a decline by 2 points postoperatively is a reliable indicator of postoperative cognitive dysfuntion (see below).

Anaesthetic techniques

Regional techniques, especially spinal analgesia, are useful in the elderly, making effective postoperative analgesia easier to achieve. Recent evidence suggests that spinal and epidural anaesthesia may decrease postoperative morbidity and mortality.

Postoperative issues

Analgesia

A misconception exists that the elderly feel less pain. Older people, however, need smaller doses of analgesic drugs to achieve effective pain relief. There is considerable variation between individuals so it is necessary to plan for each patient individually.

Postoperative cognitive dysfunction

Since 1955, it has been recognized that some elderly patients become confused and disorientated after surgery, with acute changes in personality and signs of severe anxiety and distress. Such changes have been termed postoperative cognitive disorder (POCD) (see Table 3) Patients with POCD may harm themselves, become very disruptive on the ward and may make heavy demands on nursing manpower. Occasionally, these acute personality changes can become prolonged, a situation with disastrous implications for family or carers. The reported incidence of POCD varies widely, ranging from 10–60% of patients over the age of 65.

Although a number of contributory causes for POCD have been suggested, the only proven risk factor is age itself. Evidence is accumulating that dementia in general may be caused by problems in central cholinergic pathways. So, some suggest that drugs with central anticholinergic actions such as atropine and hyoscine, phenothiazines, some antihistamines and pethidine (meperidine) should be avoided in the elderly. Pethidine has a toxic breakdown product, norpethidine, which can cause agitation and convulsions, particularly in the presence of renal impairment.

Glycopyrrolate, which does not cross the blood brain barrier, may be preferable to atropine when an anticholinergic agent is required. Pyrexia, due to wound, respiratory or urinary tract infection, and hypoxia should be eliminated as causes of acute postoperative confusion. Small doses of haloperidol, a long acting anti-psychotic, may be useful in the management of acute confusion and agitation; however, care should be taken to avoid over-sedation and the attendant risks of silent pulmonary aspiration.

High standards of nursing and medical care are vital in reducing postoperative morbidity in the elderly.

Clinical case 16

A 70-year-old patient has returned to the ward following orthopaedic surgery. The nurse is concerned that the patient is agitated and calls the house officer, who is dismissive as POCD is common. Is the house officer correct?
See comment on page 123.

The elderly

- Elderly are the fastest growing section of the population.
- Successful perioperative care in elderly requires:
  - thorough understanding of effects of ageing
  - thorough knowledge of patient's medical history
  - close supervision and monitoring.
- Polypharmacy, drug interactions and relative drug overdose are important causes of morbidity.
- Elderly tolerate fluid overload/deficit poorly.
- Postoperative cognitive dysfunction is a serious complication of anaesthesia and surgery.

Infants and children

There are marked differences between the neonate (first month of life), infant (first year of life), young child (up to 8 years), and adult. In general, the younger the child, the greater are the differences. These differences must be taken into account when caring for an infant or young child in the perioperative period (see Fig. 1).

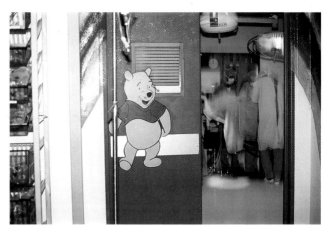

Fig. 2 **Creating a child-friendly atmosphere goes a long way towards ameliorating stress on the child and their family.**

Perioperative management

Careful preoperative assessment is pivotal to the safe practice of paediatric anaesthesia. Assessment should include evaluation of the child's current and past health, noting factors such as birth and neonatal history.

Some respiratory disorders are more common in childhood than in adult life, e.g. asthma and upper respiratory tract infections (URTIs). Mild asthma with episodes of wheezing is extremely common in young children, often associated with atopy. Severe symptoms occur in less than 10% of children and

---

CNS

- Brain and neurones develop early in intrauterine life but formation of glial cells and myelination continue during the first few years of life
- Blood–brain barrier is more permeable in the newborn period
- Nociceptive threshold may be lower than in adults

Cardiovascular

- Higher resting heart rates (i.e. newborn 90–205 bpm, infant 100–200 bpm, young child 60–140 bpm, adolescent 60–100 bpm)
- Lower systemic vascular resistance and correspondingly lower blood pressure
- Myocardial mass is less contractile (adults 60%, infants 30%) so limited ability to increase stroke volume
- Cardiac output in children is influenced more by heart rate than by stroke volume. When the tachycardia fails to maintain adequate tissue oxygenation, tissue hypoxia and hypercapnia will lead to an acidotic state and a bradycardia follows. The presence of a bradycardia in a child is a worrying sign and cardiopulmonary arrest often ensues
- Asystole tends to be more commonly observed at cardiac arrest than ventricular fibrillation

Haematopoietic

- Blood volume at birth is 90 ml/kg; adult value of 75 ml/kg by the age of 6–8 years
- At birth 75% Hb is foetal haemoglobin (HbF), but adult HbA is fully established by 6 months

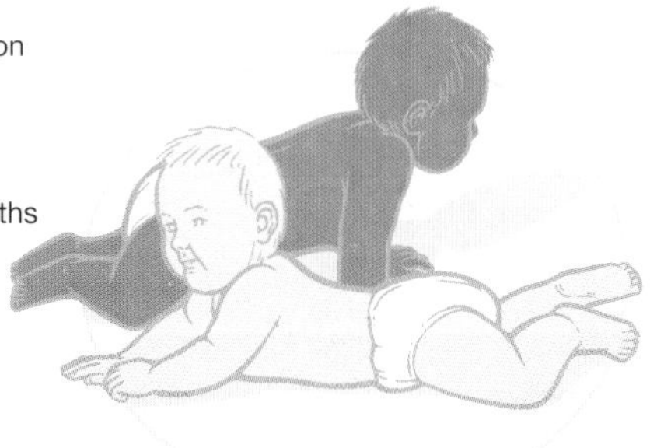

Respiratory

- Children have a high oxygen consumption at 7–8 ml/kg/min (2–3 times the adult value)
- Ventilation is almost entirely diaphragmatic
- Chest wall is more compliant
- Small airways result in high airway resistance
- Horizontally placed ribs limit ability to increase tidal or minute volume in response to demand
- Higher respiratory rate to cope with the increased oxygen consumption and carbon dioxide production
- Narrowest part of child's larynx is subglottic and not at cord level as in adults, hence the use of NON-cuffed endotracheal tubes until adolescence

Renal

- Greater proportion of body weight is water (neonate 80%, adult 60%)
- More water is extracellular than intracellular (reverse true in adults)
- Kidney function is immature at birth, glomerular filtration rate is reduced until aged 6–8 months
- Poorer ability to conserve fluid, more likely to become dehydrated with less compensate

Metabolic

- Infants and children have higher metabolic rate (about 2–3 times that of an adult)
- Liver enzymes mature rapidly after birth but detoxification and carbohydrate metabolism are poorly developed in the early neonatal period
- Synthesis of vitamin K-dependent factors (II, VII, IX, X) takes 2–3 months to mature fully
- Prone to hypoglycaemia due to poor control of glucose metabolism in the newborn, liver immaturity and low fat stores and body protein
- High surface to volume ratio increases heat loss (70% through conduction)
- Infants of less than 3 months have inadequate thermoregulatory compensatory mechanisms (e.g. little brown fat, unable to shiver)

Fig. 1 **Differences from adults which must be taken into account when caring for an infant or young child in the perioperative period.**

the majority of children have outgrown it by adolescence. Before an operation, all children should have their asthma well controlled with their usual medical regimen and be feeling well. URTIs are also common in children, with a reported frequency of 2–9 episodes each year. In a study by Cohen and Cameron in 1991, cough, laryngospasm and a decrease in oxygen saturation were reported to be increased by 2–7-fold if the child had an URTI at the time of anaesthesia and if tracheal intubation was performed such problems increased 11-fold.

Part of the preparation of the child for theatre involves recognizing and ameliorating stress experienced by the child and its family (Fig. 2). The maintenance of parental presence is to be encouraged at all ages.

Increasing numbers of operations in children are being carried out on a day-case basis, where premedication is often unnecessary. The need for premedication can further be reduced by a child-friendly atmosphere and by maintained parental presence. If a premedication is required, where possible, the oral route should be employed.

Anaesthetic implications

The anaesthetic induction period is often the most critical period for the anaesthetist as unexpected problems such as laryngospasm, bradycardia and apnoea may develop in a previously normal child. Two methods of inducing anaesthesia are routinely used in children.

Intravenous anaesthesia

Intravenous anaesthesia can be limited in children by the fact that children dislike injections. The availability and use of topical analgesia agents such as EMLA® cream and amethocaine 4% gel has made it possible to perform cannulation with the minimum of distress to the child, permitting rapid intravenous access and induction (see page 88).

Inhalation anaesthesia

The inhalational route of induction is still widely used in paediatric anaesthesia, especially in children less than 5 years-of-age. In this age group, the uptake of inhaled agents is particularly rapid. In recent years, one of the newer inhalation agents,

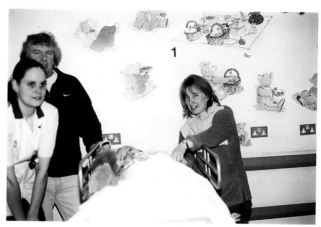

Fig. 3 **It is important to reunite parents with their children as soon as possible after the operation.**

Sevoflurane, has gained popularity as an agent for inhalational induction in children as it is relatively non-pungent and non-irritant with a high potency. Another advantage that Sevoflurane has over its older rival, Halothane, is its cardiostability and apparent lack of arrhythmogenicity.

Regional anaesthesia

Regional anaesthesia and nerve blocks are widely used in children, although mostly in conjuction with general anaesthesia. However, important differences are found in children and must be remembered when regional techniques are perfomed.

Children and especially small infants are less resistant to local anaesthetic toxicity than adults due to:

- Rapid heart rates which predisposes to bupivicaine accumulation in the heart.
- Reduced levels of α1 acid glycoprotein in neonates and infants, the protein that binds local anaesthetic.

The anatomy of the spinal cord and vertebral canal varies in the very young with the spinal cord ending at L3 compared with L2 in the adult. Ease of performance and reliability makes caudal analgesia the most commonly performed block in children. In infants and children < 2 years-of-age, due to a loose form of epidural fat, it is possible to pass an epidural catheter from the caudal entry-point up to the thoracic levels. In older children, caudal block can be used for anything surgical below the umbilicus, but as a caudal block is a major neuroaxial procedure, consideration should always be given to alternative local anaesthetic techniques (e.g. penile block for circumcision).

Postoperative care

Children should be reunited with their parents as soon as possible following their operation (Fig. 3).

Pain management and nausea and vomiting are important issues in children (see pages 98 and 68). If a child is unlikely to commence oral intake within a few hours of surgery, intravenous maintenance fluids must be established to prevent hypoglycaemia and dehydration. Hypovolaemia is the most common cause of shock in children and must be treated immediately.

Clinical case 17

An 8-year-old boy has been admitted for a tonsillectomy. What aspects of clinical practice could be implemented preoperatively to improve this boy's quality of analgesia perioperatively? Postoperatively the anaesthetist has forgotten to prescribe analgesia and you are asked to do this. What factors would you need to know before you would do this?
See comment on page 123.

Infants and children

- Infants and children are not just small adults; they differ anatomically, physiologically and in the way they handle and respond to drugs.
- Fluid balance and thermoregulation must be rigorously observed and maintained.
- Explanations appropriate for the child's age should be given before all procedures.
- Parental presence should be maintained where possible.

Pregnancy and childbirth

There are special considerations in pregnant women presenting for surgery. Normal physiological adaptations to pregnancy modify the response to stress and injury. While there are two patients to consider, until the baby is born maternal safety is the primary concern. Bleeding, pulmonary embolism and pre-eclampsia cause the majority of deaths associated with pregnancy. Specific diseases are associated with or exacerbated by pregnancy. Doctors treating pregnant women should be aware of these diseases and be familiar with their management. Surgical interventions are common during pregnancy, including caesarean sections and pregnancy terminations. Additionally, emergency surgery unrelated to pregnancy may be required.

Maternal physiological changes

Almost every organ system of the body undergoes changes (Fig. 1), which are amplified as gestation progresses and are accentuated by multiple pregnancies.

The most important changes are those affecting the cardiovascular, respiratory and haematological systems. Increased metabolic demands necessitate a pronounced increment in cardiac output, which results from increases in stroke volume and heart rate. This is accompanied by arteriolar vasodilatation leading to decreased systemic vascular resistance and mean arterial pressure. Blood pressure remains reduced until 20 weeks of gestation and then gradually rises to pre pregnancy values. When a pregnant woman lies on her back, the uterus may compress the vena cava and compromises venous return to the heart, resulting in supine hypotensive syndrome. Placing a wedge under the buttock can attenuate this.

Blood volume doubles and, despite the dilutional anaemia, moderate blood loss is well tolerated. An increase in clotting factors and fibrinogen, coupled with venous stasis, create a prothrombotic state. Surgery and bed-rest increase the risk of venous thrombosis and pulmonary embolism, and

perioperative measures aimed at preventing these complications are advisable.

Gastro-oesophageal sphincter tone and gastric emptying are decreased during pregnancy, and there is an increase in gastric secretions. These factors may render pregnant women more susceptible to aspiration of gastric contents and pulmonary injury, although there is scant evidence to support this assertion. Nonetheless, pregnant women having surgery should fast for 6–8 hours and receive a non-particulate antacid preparation prior to anaesthesia.

Foetal considerations

If surgery is deemed essential, it is best performed during the second trimester. This avoids early pregnancy when organogenesis occurs and the foetus is most vulnerable to teratogenic effects of drugs. Surgery conducted during the third trimester may precipitate preterm labour. Emergency surgery is performed throughout pregnancy with the understanding that the mother's safety is the prime concern.

Teratogenicity

Most drugs cross the placenta, with insulin and heparin being important exceptions. ACE inhibitors, alcohol, anti-epileptic drugs, tetracyclines, streptomycin, vitamin A derivatives and chemotherapy are proven teratogens. Warfarin is usually suspended during early pregnancy and replaced with heparin. Further information may be sought in the British National Formulary, which has a thorough section on prescribing in pregnancy. Most anaesthetic and analgesic agents are safe in pregnancy, although there is concern about benzodiazepines and nitrous oxide.

Pre-eclampsia

Women typically present with the syndrome of pre-eclampsia after the 20th week of pregnancy, the features of which are hypertension, proteinuria and peripheral oedema, with elevated uric acid frequently occurring. Although pre-eclampsia may be asymptomatic, in the severe or fulminant form there is hypoxic damage to maternal organ systems, as well as retarded foetal growth or death in utero. Eclampsia is a life-threatening complication of this condition, which is associated with maternal fitting. Another grave consequence of pre-eclampsia is termed HELLP syndrome (haemolysis, elevated liver enzymes and low platelets).

Management decisions are difficult in women with these pregnancy-related pathologies, as only delivery can effect cure, so maternal risk is balanced against the desire to allow pregnancy to proceed and to prevent prematurity. Eclampsia and HELLP syndrome are indications for urgent delivery. Hypertension is usually treated with methyldopa and hydralazine. Interestingly, combined data from clinical trials suggest that treatment of mild to moderate hypertension (blood pressure up to 170/110) is not beneficial and may lead to foetal growth retardation. Epidural analgesia is a useful

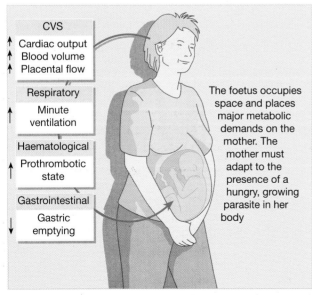

CVS
↑ Cardiac output
↑ Blood volume
↑ Placental flow

Respiratory
↑ Minute ventilation

Haematological
↑ Prothrombotic state

Gastrointestinal
↓ Gastric emptying

The foetus occupies space and places major metabolic demands on the mother. The mother must adapt to the presence of a hungry, growing parasite in her body

Fig. 1 **Physiological changes in pregnancy.**

adjunct for blood-pressure control during labour and is usually safe unless there is a severe coagulopathy or depressed level of consciousness. Central venous access and urinary catheters provide useful information about intravascular volume and fluid requirements.

These women are frequently delicately poised between developing pulmonary oedema on the one hand and renal failure on the other. Magnesium sulphate is indicated for the prevention and treatment of eclamptic fits. Admission to a high-dependency area or intensive care unit is mandatory as complications occur up to 48 hours post partum.

Haemorrhage

Extensive haemorrhage is a devastating complication of pregnancy. Abnormalities of placental location, especially placenta praevia, early placental separation or placental abruption and an abnormally adherent placenta increase the risk of bleeding. Adequate preparation before delivery, including good intravenous access, the availability of blood and the involvement of senior medical staff may avert disaster. When torrential bleeding does occur, prompt surgical intervention may prevent the evolution of a dilutional coagulopathy.

Diabetes

Diabetes mellitus and associated hyperglycaemia in the expectant mother is associated with a litany of foetal problems, including teratogenicity, macrosomia and prematurity. The end-organ damage which occurs in diabetes may be accelerated in pregnancy. Tight control of blood sugar throughout pregnancy and labour is therefore imperative and improves both neonatal and maternal outcome.

Gestational diabetes, a form of diabetes occurring during pregnancy, usually resolves following delivery. Babies born to diabetic mothers should be followed up to detect and treat hypoglycaemia.

The epidural controversy

For the expectant mother delivery is an important event, which is anticipated with emotions ranging from eagerness to trepidation. She and her partner may have preconceived ideas about the process of childbirth. There are women who want maximum involvement of medical staff and there are others who want the experience to be as natural as possible, with minimal if any medical intervention.

Doctors must be sensitive to these various views and be as accommodating as their judgement regarding patient safety allows. Information about the options for analgesia should be provided in a balanced fashion. Essentially there are four choices:

- No analgesia.
- Nitrous oxide.
- Opioid analgesia.
- Epidural analgesia (Fig. 2).

While epidural analgesia provides the best pain relief, it is unpopular with some women for various reasons. There is a perception that epidural analgesia is disempowering and is associated with several undesirable outcomes, including

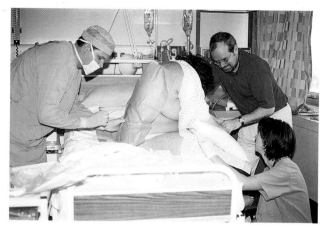
Fig. 2 **Anaesthetist inserting an epidural catheter.**

immobility, prolonged labour, chronic back pain, instrumental delivery and a high rate of caesarean section. In fact there is little evidence to support any of these views. Certainly there are complications associated with epidurals, the most important of which are failed or incomplete analgesia, and headache if the dura is punctured during epidural needle insertion. Permanent neurological injury is an exceedingly rare adverse event and occurs more frequently following traumatic passage of the baby than as a consequence of epidural analgesia. Epidural analgesia may be provided without compromising mobility and allows women to titrate pain relief to their individual requirements (Fig. 3).

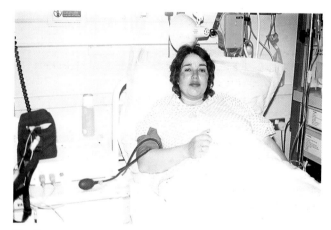
Fig. 3 **Woman in labour with a patient-controlled epidural infusion (PCEA).**

Pregnancy and childbirth

- There are two patients to consider, mother and baby.
- The most common causes of death are bleeding, pulmonary embolus and pre-eclampsia.
- Involving a multidisciplinary team increases the chance of successful outcome in high-risk pregnancies.
- Epidural analgesia is safe and does not increase the likelihood of caesarean section.

Clinical case 18

A woman presents in labour on warfarin therapy. Earlier in the pregnancy, she developed a venous thrombosis and was informed by a haematologist that she has a tendency to clot. She took her last warfarin tablet 24 hours ago. What should be done?
See comment on page 123.

Techniques of anaesthesia

The choice of anaesthetic technique depends on the type of surgery, patient risk-factors and the patient's preference. Options generally include general anaesthesia, regional anaesthesia and a combination of these techniques (Fig. 1).

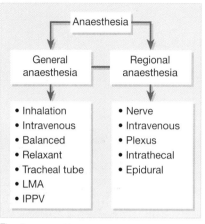

Fig. 1 **Anaesthesia options.**

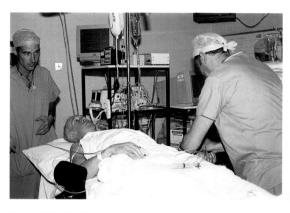

(a)

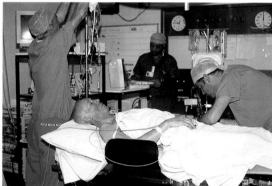

(b)

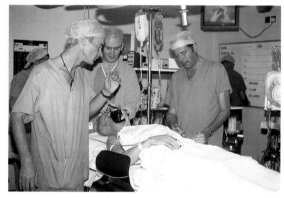

(c)

Fig. 2 **General anaesthetic sequence.**

General anaesthesia

General anaesthesia (GA) entails inducing a loss of consciousness while providing adequate operating conditions and stability of the essential physiological functions. To achieve this, the anaesthetist devises a strategy for each patient based on information acquired in a preoperative visit and knowledge of the complexity of the operation.

The induction of general anaesthesia is achieved with intravenous drugs in the majority of instances, but inhalation is a suitable alternative both for elective procedures, and in certain emergencies where the airway is compromised (see Fig. 2). Many children prefer inhalation as they are spared a needle insertion while awake. The agents used to induce anaesthesia are not always the same as for maintaining anaesthesia during surgery. The simplest general anaesthetic consists of using a single agent throughout for inducing and maintaining anaesthesia, and this can either be intravenous (using propofol) or inhalational (using sevoflurane).

Balanced anaesthesia

There is debate about whether anaesthetized patients experience pain. Strictly speaking they cannot, as they are not conscious. However, hypnotic agents alone do not prevent the responses to surgical stimuli, such as increases in blood pressure and heart rate. The addition of analgesic agents, such as opiates and non-steroidal anti-inflammatory drugs, is thought by many to be an essential component of balanced anaesthesia (see Fig. 3). The combination of general and regional anaesthesia is also a popular option. Some practitioners advocate muscle relaxants as essential ingredients in a balanced anaesthetic technique. This view is strongly opposed by those who are concerned that paralysed patients who are inadequately anaesthetized are unable to indicate that they are awake.

For sick patients, techniques with minimal depressant effects on the heart are preferable. These are based on a high dose of narcotic analgesics (such as fentanyl) and a low dose of propofol or an inhalational anaesthetic agent (such as isoflurane). If appropriate, a regional technique should be added to reduce the adrenergic response to surgery.

Emergence

Recovery from general anaesthesia depends on the elimination of agents by natural routes (lungs, liver and kidneys). Drugs with long elimination half-lives result in prolonged postoperative somnolence. Modern anaesthesia facilitates reliable hypnosis and analgesia coupled with rapid awakening and ability to function. Recent advances in anaesthetic and surgical techniques allow many operations to be carried out in day-surgery units.

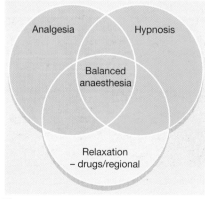

Fig. 3 **Balanced anaesthesia.**

Tracheal intubation

Placement of a tracheal tube (TT) is not a prerequisite for all patients undergoing general anaesthesia (see Fig. 4). The main indications are risk of lung soiling with gastric contents and requirement for assisted ventilation of the lungs (intermittent positive pressure ventilation – IPPV). A laryngeal mask airway (LMA) is less traumatic and better tolerated than a tracheal tube and is used during the majority of general anaesthetics in the UK (see Table 1). Positive pressure ventilation may be administered via a laryngeal mask airway when there is no pulmonary pathology.

Table 1 **Examples of clinical decision-making**

Indication	Considerations
Elective orthopaedic surgery	Regional, general or combination anaesthesia Spontaneous ventilation – LMA
Intra-thoracic surgery	Usually painful and extensive surgery – balanced anaesthetic Consider a combined regional/general anaesthetic technique Requires IPPV to inflate the lungs – tracheal intubation is necessary
Abdominal surgery	Balanced anaesthetic technique Requires muscle relaxation – tracheal intubation (or LMA) and IPPV
Liver resection	GA with low-dose hypnotic and high-dose narcotic Consider combination with epidural anaesthesia Requires muscle relaxation – tracheal intubation and IPPV

Regional anaesthesia

There is a common misconception that regional anaesthesia is safer than general anaesthesia. In reality, when performed by an experienced anaesthetist, both techniques are extremely safe. Regional anaesthesia allows the provision of excellent analgesia and decreases the need for narcotics and hypnotic drugs. There is a choice between local blocks of specific nerves or plexuses, intravenous blocks of the upper limb (Bier's), subcutaneous infiltration and neuraxial blocks.

Fig. 4 **Anaesthetized patient with a tracheal tube.**

Peripheral nerve blocks
The most commonly applied are dental nerve blocks, ocular nerve blocks for cataract surgery (see Fig. 5) and ring blocks of the fingers or toes. Other useful nerve blocks are intercostal nerve block, to alleviate pain in rib fractures or for the insertion of a chest drain and femoral nerve block for lower limb injuries.

Plexus blocks
This technique is well established for upper limb surgery (e.g. brachial plexus block) and for relief of cancer pain (e.g. coeliac plexus block).

Intravenous blocks
Intravenous blocks are used for surgery of the upper limb (Bier's block). A tourniquet is applied to the arm and a short-acting local anaesthetic agent injected through a previously inserted intravenous cannula.

Neuraxial blocks
Epidural and intrathecal blocks can be used as the sole anaesthetic for most surgery below the waistline or as an adjuvant of general anaesthesia for thoracic, abdominal, perineal and lower limb surgery. The decision to use neuraxial anaesthesia as the sole technique should be influenced by the health and the preference of the patient.

Clinical scenarios

Dental extractions
Anaesthesia for dental extraction should be provided by infiltration with local anaesthetic. The oral mucosa may be sprayed with topical lignocaine before needle insertion. General anaesthesia should be used only in exceptional circumstances, and then only in an operating theatre in an established hospital. In the UK general anaesthesia is overused for dental procedures.

Cataract surgery
Local anaesthesia avoids the risks of postoperative sedation, nausea and vomiting, and the problems introduced by cardiac and respiratory disease.

Fractured jaw after an accident
The protective laryngeal reflexes may be lost with danger of aspiration of blood, teeth and other debris. Protection of the airway is the first priority. This may be achieved by passing a tracheal tube via the nose with local anaesthesia (except when a fracture of the skull base is suspected) following which general anaesthesia may be induced.

Elderly patient for internal fixation of a hip fracture
The elderly often suffer from medical problems. The usual choice is between general anaesthesia and neuraxial block. Studies have demonstrated a reduction in blood loss and respiratory complications with such operations when performed under neuraxial blockade.

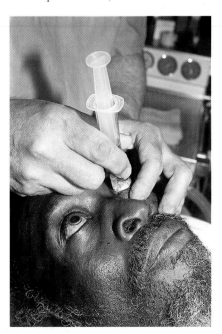

Fig. 5 **Administration of an eye block.**
Note: wearing of sherile gloves is indicated for this procedure.

> ### Techniques of anaesthesia
> - Anaesthetic techniques include general anaesthesia, regional anaesthesia and combinations of these.
> - Balanced anaesthesia entails the provision of analgesic agents in addition to hypnotic drugs.
> - Tracheal intubation is seldom essential.
> - Modern general and regional anaesthesia are extremely safe.
> - Many operations are performed in day-surgery units.

Sedation

An increasing number of minimally invasive procedures are carried out under sedation (Table 1). Such procedures are brief and cause minimal disturbance to the body's physiology, thus not justifying general anaesthesia, especially when patient cooperation is required. Sedation aims at alleviating the anxiety and discomfort associated with a procedure.

Sedation is not a discrete end-point, but lies on a continuum between complete wakefulness and general anaesthesia (Fig. 1).

Every patient responds to sedative agents differently. Sliding into general anaesthesia with loss of protective airway reflexes is an important complication of sedation. Sedative dose should be adjusted based on route of drug administration, drug interactions and patient's age and physical fitness.

Table 1 **Procedures carried out under sedation**	
Medical specialty	**Procedures**
Gastroenterology	Colonoscopy, gastroscopy
Chest medicine	Bronchoscopy
Dentistry	Extractions, root fillings, etc
Cardiology	Cardioversion, pacemaker, PTCA
Radiology	CT, MRI, etc

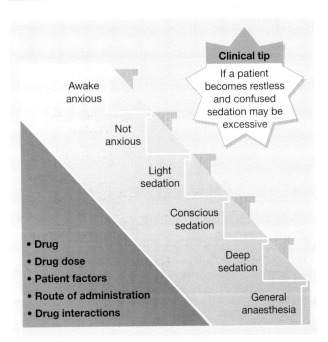

Fig. 1 **Sedation sliding scale.**

Definition

Conscious sedation is a state where the patient:

- Has a depressed level of consciousness.
- Is free from anxiety.
- Is able to protect the airway.
- Is able to respond to verbal command.

Following conscious sedation, there may be amnesia despite continuous verbal communication.

Patient selection and preoperative assessment

Appropriate patient selection reduces complications. Some patients are unsuitable for sedation and some procedures are

too long or too painful. A preoperative assessment as for general anaesthesia should be carried out.

History

In the presence of cardiac or pulmonary disease, reduced doses of sedatives may be needed. Hepatic or renal impairment may affect metabolism and excretion of sedatives leading to a longer duration of action. Previous adverse reactions to sedatives should be noted and current medication, last oral intake, and smoking or alcohol intake noted. Alcohol and smoking may increase the requirement for sedatives agents.

Examination

The airway, the lungs and the heart should be examined. Laboratory and imaging investigations are not routinely needed unless specifically indicated.

Patients must be informed about the proposed procedure and sedation plan and written consent is mandatory. Patients should be fasted 8 hours for solid foods and 2 hours for clear liquids. Inadvertent over-sedation renders patients vulnerable to regurgitation and inhalation of stomach contents. Very anxious patients may benefit from an anxiolytic medication (e.g. temazepam) given orally 2–3 hours before the procedure.

Prerequisites for safe sedation

The American Society of Anesthesiologists have issued recommendations as follows:

1) An anaesthetist should be present. It is reported in the USA that complications are less frequent when anaesthetists administer sedation. This recommendation is unlikely to be followed because there are not enough anaesthetists for the number of procedures carried out.
2) Vital signs should always be monitored. Oxygenation: the pulse oximeter is the most useful monitor. Evidence of unobstructed breathing movements should be sought throughout the period of sedation. Circulation: a non-invasive blood pressure device and an ECG monitor should be used in patients with hypertension or ischaemic heart disease. Consciousness: verbal contact with the patient should be maintained. In situations where it is not possible to speak, gestures such as 'thumbs up' can be used.

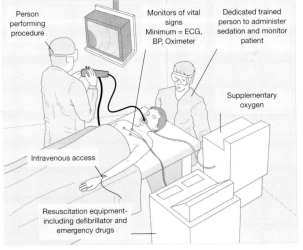

Fig. 2 **Sedation Unit set-up.**

3) The operator carrying out the procedure should not be in charge of monitoring the patient (see Fig. 2). Another member of the staff should do this. Resuscitation equipment including a defibrillator must be available.

Sedative agents

Many agents have been used for sedation, including barbiturates, chlormethiazole, antihistamine, neuroleptics, opioids, nitrous oxide, benzodiazepines and general anaesthetics. Modern sedation is based on midazolam or propofol and short-acting opioids.

Opioids

Opioids have some sedative effects but should be used only if analgesia or blunting of airway reflexes is required. Morphine, pethidine, fentanyl and remifentanil are the most widely used. Their relative potency, duration of action and side-effects differ significantly. All can induce severe ventilatory depression, nausea and vomiting, dysphoria and itching. Respiratory depression is aggravated by concurrent use of benzodiazepines. Naloxone (40–200 µg iv) is an effective competitive receptor antagonist, capable of reversing the effects of opioids. It also has severe side-effects, including pulmonary oedema.

Benzodiazepines

Benzodiazepines have important properties, inducing anxiolysis, amnesia and drowsiness. They are effective and safe and an overdose is rarely fatal. Midazolam has largely replaced diazepam; it has a shorter half-life (3 hours), causes less pain on injection and is more effective. The most serious side-effect is respiratory depression, which is more pronounced in the elderly. In an emergency, a competitive antagonist, flumazenil, is available to reverse the effects of benzodiazepines. Flumazenil is safe in a dose of 0.5–1 mg, but has a much shorter half-life than any of the benzodiazepines.

Propofol is a general anaesthetic, used for sedation in sub anaesthetic doses. It is as effective as midazolam but causes less amnesia. An advantage over the benzodiazepines is rapid recovery. Its effects can be titrated making it suitable for patient controlled sedation.

Routes of administration

- Oral and rectal routes – slow onset of action and unpredictable absorption.
- Inhalation – used in dentistry.
- Oral and nasal transmucosal – fentanyl lollipops, useful in children.
- Intramuscular – useful when veins are difficult and rapid onset is needed.
- Intravenous – rapid onset and good titration, as a bolus or as an infusion. Continuos infusion allows good intraoperative sedation and is the choice for both midazolam and propofol.

Patient-controlled sedation (PCS)

The patient may decide how much sedation is required, within certain limits (Fig. 3). The system is similar to patient controlled analgesia (PCA). The operator gives the first bolus and then the patient uses the system to maintain sedation. Propofol, with or without remifentanil, is a good choice for PCS.

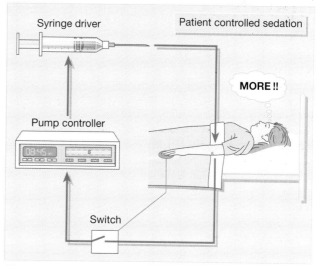

Fig. 3 **Patient-controlled sedation.**

Complications

Good patient selection and careful drug titration minimize the following complications:

- Induction of general anaesthesia may lead to airway obstruction.
- Respiratory depression results in hypoxia and hypercapnia, which cause further sedation.
- Obtunded airway reflexes increase the risk of aspiration of stomach contents, especially during gastroscopy.
- Aspiration may lead to laryngeal spasm or bronchospasm.
- Hypotension or dysrythmias.
- Agitation and disinhibition may occur paradoxically following sedation, but may be related to hypoxia or hypercarbia.

Recovery and discharge

Monitoring, particularly pulse oximetry, should be continued and vital signs recorded regularly until the patient is fully alert and orientated. If naloxone or flumazenil were given, monitoring must be continued for at least 2 hours.

In day-case surgery, the patient should be discharged into the care of a responsible adult written instructions with. Patients must not drive or operate heavy machinery until the following day.

> ### Clinical case 19
>
> A 42-year-old man requires an investigative bronchoscopy and biopsy. He is a smoker and has a body mass of 130 kg.
> *See comment on page 123–124.*

> **Sedation**
>
> - The use of sedation for surgical procedures is on the increase.
> - Effective and safe sedation is best provided by a trained anaesthetist.
> - Suitable patient selection is important.
> - Monitoring vital signs and oxygenation are essential and resuscitation equipment must be available.
> - Short-acting agents given by infusion are preferable.
> - A responsible adult should supervise patients for 24 hours.

The stress response and nutritional therapy

The stress response evolved as an adaptation to tissue injury, burns, fractures and severe infection. It is characterized by neuroendocrine responses, activation of the sympathetic nervous system and of the coagulation–fibrinolytic network (see Fig. 1). There is an acute-phase response involving cytokines and other inflammatory mediators. When an animal is injured and is threatened by acute blood loss, the physiological manifestations of the stress response increase the chance of survival, however, in the context of surgery where we inflict injury as part of an intended therapeutic intervention, certain aspects of the stress response may be deleterious.

Sympathetic activation

Sympathetic nervous system activation leads to increased oxygen requirements and may cause hypertension and myocardial ischaemia. The hormones released include cortisol, epinephrine (adrenaline), thyroid hormone, glucagon, and growth hormone, all of which increase blood glucose concentrations and induce catabolism. There is a concomitant decrease in anabolic hormones such as insulin, erthyropoietin and testosterone. Increased secretion of antidiuretic hormone leads to fluid retention and may result in hyponatraemia.

Activation of coagulation

The hypercoagulable state predisposes patients to venous thromboses, which are important causes of hospital morbidity and mortality. Inflammatory mediators and cytokines cause pain and may precipitate hyperalgesia leading to chronic pain states.

The body's response to surgery

Pain, nausea, ileus, vomiting, fatigue, sleep disturbances, hypoxia, hypothermia, pyrexia, anxiety, muscle wasting and immunosuppression are all features of the stress response to surgery. Acute-phase proteins such as C-reactive protein are released from the liver and fever often results.

There are various immunological changes associated with surgery. Macrophage and neutrophil activation is increased, whereas T cell-dependent antibody response and interferon-γ production is decreased. There is increased secretion of ACTH and leukocytosis may be present. Blood transfusion enhances postoperative immunosuppression.

Hypoxia results in decreased oxygen delivery to injured tissues and wound healing is impaired. The pain that follows surgical procedures may magnify the stress response causing a delay in restoration of function. The magnitude of the surgical stress response is related to the severity of surgical trauma.

Decreasing the stress response

If the stress response indeed represents physiological adaptation to injury, it is debatable whether we should attempt to attenuate it. Nonetheless, there is evidence that blocking some of the manifestations through targeted interventions may improve outcome. Intravenous atenolol, for example, given at the time of surgery and continued for a week, has been shown to decrease the incidence of coronary events for those at risk for up to 2 years after surgery.

Multimodal analgesia improves pain relief and may abort the development of chronic pain syndromes.

Those who have postoperative hyperglycaemia may benefit from insulin, glucose and early feeding, thus interrupting the catabolic cascade. Thrombosis prophylaxis, such as low-molecular-weight heparin and elastic stockings, should be considered for all having major surgery. Stress potentiating factors (Table 1) may be avoided in an attempt to dampen the stress response.

Neuraxial (epidural and spinal) anaesthesia with local anaesthetics almost completely abolishes the early manifestations of the stress response to surgery below the umbilicus. Neuraxial blocks decrease both intraoperative bleeding and postoperative thromboses. They are associated with less sympathetic activation and may prevent pain.

Epidural anaesthesia, initiated before surgery and maintained for 48 hours post-surgery, prevents the decrease in protein synthesis and the increase in protein degradation that is typically seen with surgical stress.

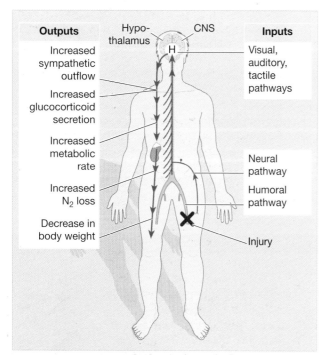

Fig. 1 **The stress response.**

Table 1 **Factors potentiating the stress response**
Anxiety and fear
Pain
Handling of viscera
Tissue injury
Blood loss and absorption of haematoma
Dehydration and starvation
Hypothermia
Hypxoxia and hypercarbia
Bacteraemia and release of bacterial toxins
Anaphylactic and anaphylactoid reactions

High-dose opioids may blunt the stress response, but do not prevent it. Minimally invasive surgical procedures, such as the use of laparascopic techniques, may modify the surgical stress response. There is a subsequent reduction in protein catabolism, inflammatory mediators, pulmonary dysfunction and convalescence.

Prevention of intraoperative heat loss decreases the stress response, the wound infection rate and possibly even cardiovascular complications. Cytokine antagonists, free radical scavengers, glucocortcoids and other anti-inflammatory agents have been suggested as potential modifiers of the stress response. Neostigmine has recently been shown to be useful for the treatment of postoperative pseudo-obstruction and ileus.

It is extremely difficult to achieve stress-free anaesthesia and surgery. Yet, in striving to do so, we may hope to decrease an assortment of postoperative complications. Minimally invasive surgery may constitute an important step in this direction.

Starvation and catabolism

In the surgical patient, the stress response coupled with the decreased intake of food leads to considerable weight loss. The patient may lose up to 30 g of nitrogen per day. In simple starvation (non-surgical), blood glucose concentration falls, and the patient only loses about 5–10 g of nitrogen a day. While providing nutrition may reverse simple starvation, the catabolism following surgery may be refractory to attempts at maintaining energy intake.

Maintaining a normal food intake preoperatively and providing early postoperative nutrition improves wound healing and reduces catabolism considerably.

Oral dietary supplements

Whenever possible, oral or enteral feeding should be instituted. If the patient is able to eat, then diet can be supplemented with defined liquid formulae. Milk based formulae are more palatable, but are not suitable for patients with lactose intolerance. Milk free formulae can be elemental (free amino acids), semi-elemental (small peptides) and polymeric (whole protein). Lactose free polymeric formulae (Ensure®, Osmolite®) are commonly used and are iso-osmolar drinks containing 1 kcal/ml as 16% protein, 55% carbohydrate and 30% fat.

Enteral feeding

Enteral feeding is used when the patient cannot or will not ingest adequate nutrients. Short term (< 6 weeks anticipated) tube feeding can be achieved by placement of a soft, small bore nasogastric or nasojejunal feeding tube (Fig. 2). Agents to improve gastric motility, such as metoclopromide and erythromycin, may be administered. A postpyloric tube allows

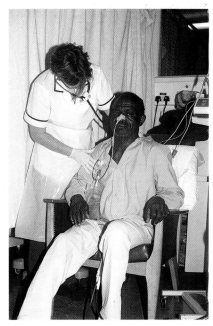

Fig. 2 **Patient with a nasogastric tube.**

enteral feeding despite gastric stasis. Long-term (> 6 weeks) tube feeding usually requires placement of a gastrostomy or jejunostomy tube. Commonly the tube is placed endoscopically (percutaneous endoscopic gastrostomy, PEG). Feeding schedules can be intermittent or continuous. During and for 2 hours after bolus intermittent feeds, the patient's upper body should be elevated. Complications of enteral feeding include tube misplacement, erosive tissue damage from the tube, tube occlusion, pulmonary aspiration of feeds, and diarrhoea.

Total parenteral nutrition (TPN)

The intestinal tract cannot be used in patients with persistent nausea and vomiting, intolerable postprandial abdominal pain or diarrhoea, mechanical obstruction, severe hypomotility, malabsorbtion or high output fistulae. In general, TPN should be considered when energy intake has been or is anticipated to be inadequate (<50% of daily requirement) for more than 7 days and enteral feeding is not possible. TPN is administered through a central venous catheter. Peripherally inserted central catheters (PICC) can also be used. Macronutrient solutions containing crystalloid amino acid solutions, glucose and lipid emulsion are infused at a rate of approximately 0.05g/Kg/hour. The complications of TPN are reduced with careful management and close supervision. Typical problems include pneumothorax and carotid artery puncture during line placement, fluid overload, refractory hyperglycaemia, electrolyte derangement, hypertriglyceridaemia, pulmonary embolism and thrombosis, catheter related sepsis and deranged liver function.

Clinical case 20

A 66-year-old man has returned to the ward following a laparatomy for bowel cancer. He complains of pain (despite regular morphine injections), feeling bloated and nausea. Tympanic temperature is 34.7°C, blood glucose is 14 mmol/l and urine output is 20 ml/hour. His abdomen is distended and there are no bowel sounds. What measures might be taken to decrease morbidity and the risk of postoperative complications?
See comment on page 124.

The stress response

- Certain aspects of the body's response to injury or the stress response may be deleterious following surgery.

- Epidural analgesia decreases the stress response to surgical procedures below the umbilicus.

- Minimally invasive surgery represents an important advance.

- Early enteral feeding is beneficial following surgery.

Antibiotic prophylaxis

The risk of developing a surgical site infection (SSI) appears to be a balance between patient-related factors, microbial factors and wound-related factors (Fig. 1).

Patient-related factors

Chronic illness, extremes of age or immunocompromise including diabetes mellitus and corticosteroid therapy are associated with an increased risk of developing SSI. The American Society of Anesthesiologists (page 7) score of 3 or more, indicative of a patient in poor medical condition, when combined with the type and duration of surgery has been shown to be predictive of the rate of SSI.

Microbial factors

Enzyme production (*Staphylococcus aureus*), possession of polysaccharide capsule (*Bacteroides fragilis*) and the ability to bind to fibronectin in blood clots (*S. aureus* and *Staphylococcus epidermidis*) are mechanisms by which microorganisms exploit weakened host defences and initiate infection. Biofilm formation, exemplified by *S. epidermidis*, is particularly important in the aetiology of prosthetic material infections e.g. prosthetic joint infection

Wound-related factors

Devitalized tissue, dead space, and haematoma formation are factors associated with the development of SSI. Historically, wounds have been described as clean, contaminated and dirty according to the expected number of bacteria entering the surgical site (Table 1).

Prophylactic antimicrobials

The administration of antimicrobial prophylaxis for surgery has been shown to decrease greatly the incidence of postoperative infection, particularly where the inoculum of bacteria is high,

(Fig. 2). The presence of a foreign body (such as sutures) reduces the inoculum required to induce SSI from 10^6–10^2 organisms.

such as in colonic or vaginal surgery, or where there is insertion of an artificial device, for example, a hip prosthesis or heart valve.

Spectrum of antibiotics

Broadly speaking, infections associated with clean surgery are caused by Staphylococcal species and infections of contaminated suregry are polymicrobial in origin and comprise the flora of the viscus entered (e.g. *Esherichia. coli* and *B. fragilis* in colonic surgery). The antibacterial spectrum, low incidence of side-effects and tolerability of cephalosporins have made them the ideal choice for prophylaxis (Table 2).

The increasing prevalence of both methicillin-resistant *Staphylococcus aureus* (MRSA), against which cephalosporins are ineffective and *Clostridium difficile*-associated diarrhoea, a disorder associated with

Table 1 Classification criteria of operative wounds according to level of bacterial contamination

Classification criteria	Description	Typical infection rates (%)
Clean wound	Non-traumatic, not inflamed, hollow viscus not entered	1–3
Clean–contaminated wound	Non-traumatic, entry of hollow viscus or mucous membrane surface with minimal spillage of contents	8–10
Contaminated wound	Fresh traumatic wound, entry of hollow viscus with spillage, especially colon. Operative site contaminated by infected bile or urine, acute inflammation present	15–20
Dirty wound	Old traumatic wound with devitalized tissue, presence of foreign body, faecal contamination or existing infection	25–40

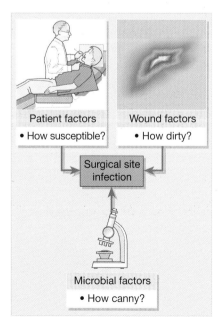

Fig. 1 **Factors predisposing to surgical site infection.**

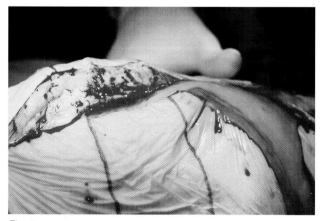

Fig. 2 **Surgical site infection associated with recent implantation of a prosthetic hip.**

Table 2 Antibiotic prophylaxis regimens for common surgical procedures (NB policy may vary according to the local situation)

System	Surgery	Antibiotic regime
Gastrointestinal	Upper bowel and biliary	Cefuroxime 750 mg iv
	Large bowel and appendix	Cefuroxime 750 mg + metronidazole 500 mg iv
	ERCP	Ciprofloxacin 750 mg po
Orthopaedics	Simple open fracture	Cefuroxime 750 mg iv
	Joint replacement and internal fixations	Cefuroxime 750 mg iv, 8-hourly for 24 hours
Gynaecological	Hysterectomy	Cefuroxime 750 mg + metronidazole 500 mg iv
	Caesarean section	Cefuroxime 750 mg iv after the cord is clamped
Urinary tract	TURP and cystoscopy	Ciprofloxacin 500 mg po

cephalosporin use, may result in the substitution of other agents in future.

Timing

The 'decisive period' is 0–2 hours before surgery. Three hours after surgical incision, prophylaxis is no longer effective.

Duration

For most procedures a single dose is adequate. Prolonged surgery (> 3 hours) may necessitate a second dose. Prophylaxis should certainly be discontinued within 24 hours of the procedure.

Prosthetic devices

Prophylaxis is given for 24 hours.

Dirty surgery

Antibiotics are given therapeutically as full courses (5–7 days), e.g. bowel perforation, complex open fracture.

Skull fractures

The literature does not support the use of prophylactic antimicrobials in closed skull fractures with or without CSF leakage. Antibiotic use may select resistant flora.

MRSA

During an outbreak or when methicillin-resistant *Staphylococcus aureus* (MRSA) is endemic in the ward, vancomycin or teicoplanin prophylaxis should be used in cardiac, vascular and orthopaedic surgery.

Table 3 Procedures for which prophylaxis for endocarditis is recommended

Dental procedures
Respiratory procedures
Tonsillectomy
Surgery involving respiratory mucosa
Rigid bronchoscopy
Gastrointestinal procedures
Sclerotherapy of varices
Oesophageal dilatation
ERCP
Biliary tract surgery
Surgery involving intestinal mucosa
Genitourinary procedures
Prostatic surgery
Cystoscopy
Urethral dilatation

Infective endocarditis prophylaxis

Certain surgical procedures (Table 3) are associated with bacteraemia, which puts patients with certain cardiac abnormalities at risk of infective endocarditis (IE). Antibiotic prophylaxis is indicated in such cases (see Table 4).

The main cardiac indications are rheumatic heart disease, prosthetic heart valves, congenital heart disease, mitral valve prolapse with regurgitation, a previous episode of IE, and hypertrophic obstructive cardiomyopathy. Patients at particularly high risk are those with a prosthetic heart valve or a history of IE.

Antibiotic prophylaxis is not indicated in patients with coronary artery disease, previous bypass surgery or permanent pacemakers.

Clinical case 21

A patient who is aged 67 years and has mitral stenosis after rheumatic fever as a child is undergoing a colonoscopy for chronic diarrhoea. Is antibiotic prophylaxis indicated? *See comment on page 124.*

Antibiotic prophylaxis

- Antibiotic prophylaxis if given appropriately is very effective.
- In the pathogenesis of surgical site infection (SSI) there is a balance between host defences, microbial virulence and wound factors.
- Wounds can be prognostically classified as being clean, clean–contaminated, contaminated or dirty.
- Timing – the 'decisive period' is thought to be 0–2 hours before surgery.
- Duration – prophylaxis should be discontinued within 24 hours of the procedure.
- Dirty surgery – antibiotics are given therapeutically as full courses (5–7 days).
- MRSA – requires the use of vancomycin/teicoplanin prophylaxis in cardiac, vascular and orthopaedic surgery.
- Prevention of bacterial endocarditis should be priority. A risk-assessment should be made on each case.

Table 4 Suggested regimens for the prophylaxis of infective endocarditis (NB policy may vary according to the local situation)

Indication	Dosage	Timing
Standard general prophylaxis	Amoxicillin 3.0 g po	1 hour prior to procedure
	Amoxicillin 1.5 g po	6 hours after
Unable to take oral medication	Ampicillin 2.0 g iv or im	30 min prior to procedure
Allergic to penicillin	Clindamycin 600 mg po, or cephalexin 2.0 g po, or azithromycin or clarithromycin 500 mg po	1h prior to procedure
Allergic to penicillin, unable to take oral	Clindamycin, adults 600 mg iv, or cefazolin 2.0 g iv or im, or vancomycin 1 g iv	30 min prior to procedure
Gastrointestinal or genitourinary procedures	Gentamicin 1.5 mg/kg iv or im should be added to regimen	

Fluid management

Water is the major constituent of the human body, composing 60–80% of total body mass (Fig. 1). Body water is distributed in three compartments. About 60% of the water is intracellular and 40% is extracellular, of which 75% is interstitial fluid and 25% is intravascular (Fig. 2). The blood volume in adults is usually 5–6 litres. The average person has minimum obligatory daily fluid losses exceeding a litre and typically requires a daily fluid intake of about 2.5 litres.

There is significant fluid flux in the perioperative period. Patients presenting for surgery frequently have a fluid deficit, having been nil by mouth for at least 8 hours. This fluid deprivation is unnecessary as it is both safe and desirable to have unlimited clear fluids

Table 1	**Features of hypervolaemia and hypovolaemia**	
	Hypovolaemia	**Hypervolaemia**
Suggestive history	Thirst, exercise, oliguria, blood loss, burns, trauma, diarrhoea and vomiting, diabetes, polyuria, diuretic therapy, orthostatic syncope, infection	Intravenous fluid therapy, heart failure, kidney failure, liver failure
Suggestive clinical signs	Dry mucous membranes, sunken eyes, tachycardia, orthostatic hypotension, pulsus paradoxus, thready pulse, decreased skin turgor, confusion, concentrated urine, decreased body mass, cold peripheries with poor capillary refill	Peripheral oedema, ascites, elevated jugular venous pulsation (JVP), basal lung crackles, confusion, sweating, increased body mass
Suggestive investigations	High urine osmolaliy, low urine output, high plasma urea, no increase in JVP and wedge pressure to fluid challenge, decreased cardiac output, swings in pressure trace of pulse oximeter and arterial line, decreased end tidal CO_2	Low urine osmolality, high urine output, low plasma urea, exaggerated increase in JVP and wedge pressure to fluid challenge, evidence of cardiomegaly and pulmonary oedema on CXR, echocardiographic evidence of increased cardiac filling
Possible problems	Decreased venous return to the heart and hypovolaemic shock Prerenal failure progressing to established renal failure Vital organ hypoperfusion resulting in ischaemic cerebral, myocardial, renal, and liver injury Inadequate tissue oxygenation leading to anaerobic metabolism and lactic acidosis	Cardiac failure Cerebral oedema and raised intracranial pressure, which may cause irreversible brain damage Pulmonary oedema causing intrapulmonary shunting leading to hypoxaemia and all its attendant problems Impaired oxygen delivery at a tissue level

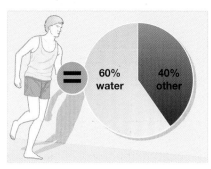

Fig. 1 **Water composition of the human body.**

up to 2 hours before elective surgery. Some patients are at risk for profound dehydration, including those who have lost excessive volume through blood, urine, sweat, faeces or vomitus. Dehydration may be prevented in these circumstances through early administration of sufficient and appropriate intravenous fluids.

During surgery obligatory fluid losses through urine (measured losses), sweating and breathing (insensible losses) continue. Additionally there is bleeding and third-space losses (sequestration of fluid into tissues, gastrointestinal tract and peritoneal space). Fluid losses are ongoing in the postoperative period. Throughout this time, patients are unable to fulfil their own fluid requirements and it falls to medical and nursing staff to provide adequate resuscitation.

Antidiuretic hormone and mineralocorticoids are released as part of the stress response to surgery. Urine output cannot thus be relied upon for evaluation of intravascular volume, although output persistently less than 0.5 ml/kg/hour is worrying. Not surprisingly, both hypovolaemia and fluid overload are common perioperative complications necessitating regular clinical assessment and accurate monitoring of fluid balance (Table 1).

Perioperative fluid requirements

Deficit and maintenance

Maintenance fluid requirements can be estimated as 1.5 ml/kg/hour or more conservatively as 1 ml/kg/hour when fluid restriction is indicated. Maintenance fluids, 5% dextrose being a

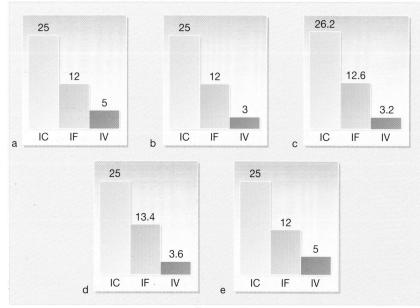

Fig. 2 **Body fluid distribution. (a)** Average 70 kg adult male. **(b)** Following 2 l acute blood loss. **(c)** Replacement of acute blood loss with 5% dextrose. **(d)** Replacement of acute blood loss with crystalloid. **(e)** Replacement of acute blood loss with colloid (IC = intracellular fluid, IF = interstitial fluid, IV = intravascular fluid).

typical example, are administered to replace insensible losses from all three body compartments. Dextrose solutions are not good plasma volume expanders because the dextrose is metabolized and water distributes freely into all compartments. Pure water is not administered via the intravenous route, as it would flood into red cells and cause haemolysis.

In addition to obligatory water loss, there is concomitant electrolyte loss, particularly sodium, chloride, potassium and magnesium. For acute deficit and replacement it is usually necessary to administer fluids containing only sodium and chloride, as these are the most abundant extracellular ions. If sodium is not given, life-threatening hyponatraemia may result. An adult needs about 9 g of sodium daily. 0.9% saline (normal saline) contains 0.9 g of sodium chloride per 100 ml of water, or 9 g per litre, enough for daily salt requirements.

Excessive fluid replacement therapy with chloride-containing compounds may result in hyperchloraemia and metabolic acidosis. In order to avoid this it is sometimes appropriate to use solutions with lower chloride than sodium concentrations, such a Ringer-Lactate (Hartmann's solution).

Replacement

Acute fluid losses deplete plasma volume more rapidly than other body compartments. Replacement should be with fluids which stay in the extracellular space. Balanced salt solutions (normal saline, Ringer's lactate), colloids and blood products satisfy this requirement. There is no evidence that colloids improve survival compared with crystalloids following acute losses (see Fig. 3).

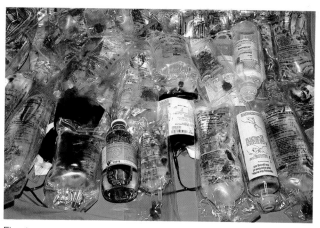
Fig. 4 **Which fluid when?**

Acute fluid loss occurs with haemorrhage, burns, pancreatitis, peritonitis, diarrhoea, ileus and losses from the upper gastrointestinal tract. In sepsis, profound vasodilation coupled with loss of fluid into the interstitium results in intravascular hypovolaemia.

Blood loss should be replaced initially with a crystalloid solution (balanced salt solution) with a volume of three times the blood loss, as the crystalloid will distribute throughout the extracellular space. 2 litres of warmed Ringer-lactate is frequently the initial fluid resuscitation following major trauma. Subsequent replacement of blood loss may be with a colloid solution, which is temporarily confined to the plasma space (see Fig. 2).

Crystalloid administration may increase the risks of fluid overload and intersitial oedema (see Fig. 2). Colloids, on the other hand, will leak into the interstitial space within several hours and may cause platelet dysfunction. All patients who receive large amounts of fluids may develop a dilutional coagulopathy.

Debate rages about the most appropriate fluid in a given setting (Fig. 4). There is little evidence in the medical literature to provide reliable guidance. Currently, many doctors choose a judicious mixture of crystalloids and colloids. Starch and gelatine based colloids are popular because, theoretically, they remain in the plasma compartment longer. Albumin has become less popular owing to cost and evidence suggesting that in certain groups of patients, albumin administration may be associated with increased mortality.

Clinical case 22

A previously healthy 55-year-old man with a body mass of 80 kg has undergone major colonic surgery for cancer. Intraoperative fluid therapy was appropriate and the haemoglobin was 11 g/dl following surgery. If he is expected to lose 500 ml of blood over the next 24 hours and is unable to take oral fluids, write an appropriate fluid chart for his needs.
See comment on page 124.

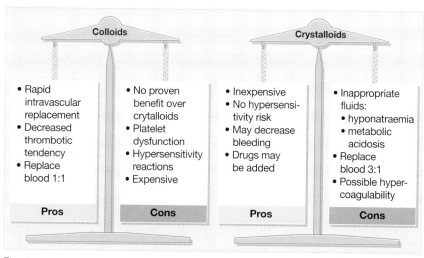

Colloids		Crystalloids	
Pros	**Cons**	**Pros**	**Cons**

• Rapid intravascular replacement
• Decreased thrombotic tendency
• Replace blood 1:1
	• No proven benefit over crytalloids
	• Platelet dysfunction
	• Hypersensitivity reactions
	• Expensive
		• Inexpensive
		• No hypersensitivity risk
		• May decrease bleeding
		• Drugs may be added
			• Inappropriate fluids:
			  • hyponatraemia
			  • metabolic acidosis
			• Replace blood 3:1
			• Possible hyper-coagulability

Fig. 3 **The pros and cons of colloids and crystalloids.**

Fluid management

- Hypervolaemia and hypovolaemia are common perioperative problems.

- Fluid therapy should aim to replace fluid deficit, insensible losses and acute losses.

- A pure dextrose solution may be administered to replace some of the insensible water loss, but does not replace electrolytes and is unsuitable for acute losses.

- Dangerous hyponatraemia may result if dextrose solutions are administered exclusively.

- Balanced salt solutions and colloids are suitable for acute resuscitation.

Blood products

Life is unsustainable without the constant flow of blood. Every minute the total blood volume circulates throughout the body. Nutrients, hormones and drugs are delivered in the blood to the various organ systems, and waste products are collected and couriered to the lungs, kidneys and liver for disposal. Haemoglobin is a specialized molecule in red blood cells, whose designated task is the efficient carriage of oxygen. When the body is threatened by infection, white cells, macrophages, cytokines, complement, killer cells and immunoglobulins meet the onslaught. Platelets and clotting factors are adapted to plug breeches and promote coagulation, thereby preventing exsanguination following injury.

Transfusion

Healthy volunteers donate whole blood, which is fractionated into packed (red blood) cells, plasma, cryoprecipitate and platelets (see Table 1). These components may be life-saving when infused into the bloodstream of recipients who have inadequate haemoglobin levels, impaired platelet function or clotting disorders. Immunoglobins and specific clotting factors are also obtained from donor blood.

Changes in transfusion practice

The term 'transfusion trigger' is used to denote the circumstances when transfusion would be reasonable. For many years it was advocated that surgical patients should receive a blood transfusion if the haemoglobin fell below 10 g/dl or if the haematocrit dropped below 30%, the '10/30 rule'. Blind adherence to this rule resulted in countless unnecessary blood transfusions with the attendant complications and costs.

No single laboratory value should be used as a trigger, rather several factors should be considered. These include age, underlying medical conditions, type and time-course of the anaemia, amount of anticipated blood loss and the presence of lactic acidosis or hypoxaemia. Even for critically ill patients, evidence suggests that transfusion may be withheld if the haemoglobin exceeds 8 g/dl. Treatment with haematinics or recombinant erythropoietin increases haemoglobin concentration and may subvert the need for transfusion.

Fresh frozen plasma (FFP) is frequently transfused inappropriately, with many doctors administering plasma whenever there is significant blood loss. In reality, only a fraction of normal clotting factor concentration is needed for adequate coagulation. FFP is indicated only if clotting tests confirm a coagulopathy. Empirical transfusion may be warranted if there has been massive blood loss (more than twice the blood volume) with inadequate haemostasis.

Platelet transfusion is usually indicated if the platelet count is less than $50 \times 10^9/L$ at the time of major surgery or if there is documented platelet dysfunction. Aspirin therapy is not an indication for platelet transfusion. The effects on operative bleeding of newer anti-platelet drugs, like clopidogrel, ticlopidine and abciximab, are not well established. Thrombocytopenia and impaired platelet function are more common than clotting factor deficiencies following major trauma and surgery.

Collection and storage

Blood products are screened for antibodies to Hepatitis B and C viruses, human immunodeficiency virus and syphilis.

Red blood cells are stored in bags containing additives and anticoagulant. Typical additive solutions are SAG-M (sodium chloride, adenine, glucose and mannitol) with citrate and CPD-A (citrate, phosphate, dextrose, adenine). The sugar, phosphate and adenine provide energy for the cells and render them viable for up to 35 days if stored at 4–6°C. Phosphate is added in an attempt to preserve 2,3 DPG levels in stored red cells. Depletion of 2,3 DPG reduces offloading of oxygen from haemoglobin by shifting the oxyhaemoglobin dissociation curve to the left. Citrate is an anticoagulant, which is rapidly metabolized by the liver following transfusion.

Platelets are stored at 22°C only for 5 days because of the risk of bacterial contamination. Plasma separated from whole blood may be rapidly frozen and stored at –30°C. Thawing FFP at 4°C and then refreezing to –30°C yields cryoprecipitate. Blood products in the UK are leukocyte-depleted to reduce the occurrence of febrile non-haemolytic reactions, as well as possibly reducing the transmission of prion disease, variant – Creutzveldt–Jacob.

Pretransfusion tests

Before transfusion, a sample of the patient's blood must be collected and the blood group determined. The ABO and Rhesus groups are of major clinical significance, since antibodies to donor red cells can cause fatal transfusion reactions.

The patient's blood is tested for red cell antibodies and is mixed with the donor red cells (cross-match) to ensure compatibility. The bedside check of patient identity against the blood units is vital to prevent fatal errors (Fig. 1). Two health professionals, both of whom

Table 1	**Blood components and their uses.**
Component	**Uses**
Whole blood	Acute, large-volume bleed
	Exchange transfusion
Packed red cells	Symptomatic anaemia
	Major acute blood loss
Platelets	Thromboctyopenia with bleeding
	Massive transfusion with dilutional coagulopathy and active bleeding
	Platelet dysfunction (congenital or acquired) with bleeding
Fresh frozen plasma	Emergency correction of acquired and inherited coagulation defects
	Massive blood transfusion with bleeding
	Emergency reversal of warfarin therapy
	Liver failure with bleeding
Cryoprecipitate	Low fibrinogen levels

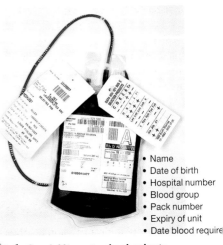

- Name
- Date of birth
- Hospital number
- Blood group
- Pack number
- Expiry of unit
- Date blood require

Fig. 1 **Crucial items to check prior to administering blood.**

Table 2 **Complications of blood transfusion**

Acute complications	Cause	Comments
Haemolytic transfusion reaction (mismatch)	ABO incompatibility	Usually due to clerical and administrative errors
		10% mortality
Febrile non-haemolytic reaction	Antileukocyte antibodies	Decreased with leukocyte-depleted blood
Urticaria	Antibodies to infused plasma proteins	
Anaphylaxis	As for urticaria	
Transfusion-related acute lung injury (TRALI)	Donor plasma has antibodies to patient's leukocytes	May be fatal
		Occurs with massive transfusion
Dilutional coagulopathy	Massive transfusion	
Septic shock	Bacterial contamination of blood products	
Congestive cardiac failure	Volume overload	
Hypothermia		Warm blood if large volume transfused
Hyperkalaemia		Usually transient
Hypocalcaemia		Usually transient
Citrate toxicity	Massive transfusion	Treat with iv calcium chloride
Delayed complications		
Delayed haemolytic transfusion reaction	Antibodies to donor red cell antigens which are not detected in the cross-match	
Graft versus host disease	Donor T cell response against immunodeficient recipient	Often fatal
Immunosuppression	Related to white cell exposure	Cancer recurrence and postoperative infection
Viral infection	Failure to detect virus in donor blood	Risk depends on virus:
		HIV < 1 in 3 × 10^6; HBV/HCV < 1 in 200 000
Iron overload	Multiple transfusions	

sign that they have checked the blood before transfusion, must perform the check. In emergencies when there is insufficient time to wait for cross-matched blood, group O Rhesus-negative blood may be given. Specific compatibility is not necessary for plasma, which is pooled from multiple donors, or platelets, which may be pooled or from a single donor.

Complications of transfusions

The complications of red cell transfusions are shown in Table 2. The major risk with plasma and platelets is infection. Following a platelet transfusion, patients develop antibodies to platelet antigens. There is a high risk of thrombocytopenia with a subsequent platelet transfusion. If a high volume is transfused there is a danger of hypothermia unless the blood is warmed (Fig. 2).

Alternatives to homologous transfusion

Autologous blood transfusion involves the use of the patient's own blood, thereby avoiding several of the hazards of blood transfusion. However donation prior to surgery is generally not considered cost-effective. Acute normovolaemic haemodilution entails removal of blood at the start of surgery and simultaneous replacement with crystalloid or colloid. This lowers haematocrit so that fewer red cells are lost. Collected blood, rich in cells and clotting factors, is transfused following surgery. Intraoperative blood salvage systems have been developed, which allow collection and re-infusion of blood during surgery. Red cell substitutes offer an alternative to blood transfusion, but are currently expensive and of limited efficacy.

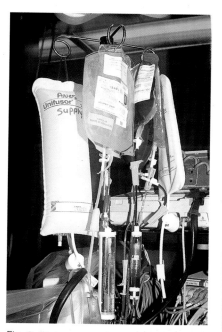

Fig. 2 **Patients during and after surgery may receive massive transfusions of blood and blood products with all their attendant complications.**

Clinical case 23

A patient receiving a blood transfusion on the ward develops pyrexia of 38.3°C and the heart rate increases to 110 beats/min. The patient complains of sweating and mild itching. What should be done?
See comment on page 124.

Blood products

- Whole blood is rarely required.
- Packed red cell transfusion is seldom indicated when the haemoglobin exceeds 8 g/dl.
- There are numerous complications associated with blood transfusion.
- Two health professionals should check blood before it is administered.
- Empirical transfusion of platelets and FFP should be avoided.

Oximetry and capnography

The pulse oximeter provides a continuous, non-invasive, indirect in vivo measurement of the proportion of oxyhaemoglobin to total haemoglobin in arterial blood. It estimates the oxygenation of arterial blood, thus replacing invasive measurements of PaO_2 in samples of arterial blood. The pulse oximeter has become indispensable for monitoring patients receiving sedation or anaesthesia and for those in the intensive care unit.

Pulse oximetry was developed following a chance observation in 1971 that arterial pulsations (observed in two signals received from an ear oximeter transmitting light at 805 and 900 nm) showed a change in relative amplitude during breath-holding. It took another 15 years to develop a device for clinical use and for its acceptance in routine clinical monitoring.

Pulse oximeters display *functional saturation* in %, which represents the proportion of oxyhaemoglobin in the sum of oxy- and reduced haemoglobin according to the equation

$$Sat\,(\%) = \frac{100 \times HbO_2}{(HbO_2 + Hb\text{-red})}$$

Oximetry

At 660 nm (red) and 940 nm (infra-red) light absorption coefficients are different for haemoglobin and oxyhaemoglobin allowing the measurement of the relative amounts of the two states. Two additional beams of different wavelengths are needed to measure methaemoglobin or carboxy-haemoglobin. Standard bench oximeters measure absorption at 4 or more wavelengths.

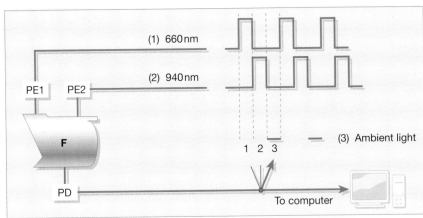

Fig. 2 **Diagram of the pulse oximeter**. F = finger, PE = light-emitting diodes, PD = photodiode. The output of the detector responds in sequence to the two light-emitting diodes and to ambient light.

Pulse oximetry

Pulse oximeters use beams at 660 and 940 nm. A finger probe (see Fig. 1) contains two light-emitting diodes on one side of the finger and a single photodiode on the other, to pick up the radiation transmitted through the tissue. Each diode emits short pulses of light and the frequency of switching between the two wavelengths is very rapid (> 400 Hz). Between the light pulses there is a short interval without emission when the detector picks up ambient light in order to subtract this signal (see Fig. 2).

The pattern of the signal in a finger probe is in Fig. 3. There are two components of the signal: a steady component arising from the non-vascular parts of the tissue, the venous blood and non-pulsatile arterial blood, and a pulsatile component, typically 2% of the steady one, arising from the alternating filling and emptying of the arterioles with each cardiac pulsation. Its amplitude depends on the arterial pressure wave and on the proportion of oxyhaemoglobin. A decrease in oxyhaemoglobin leads to a decrease in amplitude of the pulsatile signal picked up from the 940 nm diode and an increase in that from the 660 nm diode.

Pulse oximeters have an integral computer which first calculates the ratios between the pulsatile and steady components of the signals at 660 and 940 nm, and then the ratio between these two ratios is calculated. The final reading in % results from a complex calculation following an algorithm derived from simultaneous measurements made in a bench oximeter during hypoxic experiments in volunteers. All pulse oximeters are calibrated at the factory empirically. Accuracy varies from instrument to instrument and values of less than 60% are unreliable.

Several factors can cause false readings or prevent pulse oximeters from functioning:

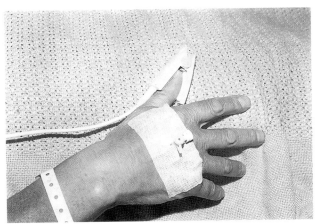

Fig. 1 **Pulse oximeter finger probe in situ perioperatively.**

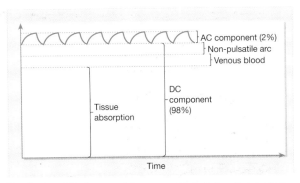

Fig. 3 **Simplified trace of the reconstituted signal picked up by the photodiode of a pulse oximeter at one wavelength.**

- Methaemoglobinaemia and carboxyhaemoglobin cause over-estimation errors. Fetal Hb and hyperbilirubinaemia do not interfere with readings.
- Artefact – poor peripheral perfusion (hypovolaemia, hypothermia, left ventricular failure or compression of supplying arteries by BP cuff) results in a poor pulsatile signal and unreliable or unobtainable reading.
- Artefact – movement of the probe or of the limb where the probe is applied may cause erroneous readings, especially if the movement is rhythmic.

Most pulse oximeters alert the user to a poor signal, meaning that the pulsatile fraction of the light received is less than 0.5% of total light; the machine alerts the user to the unreliability of the reading.

Capnography

Capnography is the measurement of carbon dioxide (CO_2) in respiratory gases (see Fig. 4). It is a very useful monitor for patients under anaesthesia and for those in intensive care units for the following reasons:

- It indicates if the lungs are being ventilated (can be linked to an alarm).
- It excludes oesophageal placement of a tracheal tube.
- End-tidal CO_2 can be used as a guide to adjust mechanical ventilation.
- Short-term variations in end-tidal CO_2 indicate variations in cardiac output

or sharp changes in metabolic rate (e.g. malignant hyperthermia).
- Variations in the shape of the capnograph waveform indicate changes in dead space (e.g. in pulmonary gas embolism) or maldistribution of ventilation (e.g. in bronchospasm).

The most commonly used capnograph uses the infra-red light absorption property of CO_2 to measure its concentration. The main components of air (nitrogen and oxygen) do not absorb infra-red light. Gases and vapours used in anaesthesia (nitrous oxide, isoflurane) absorb infra-red light with a characteristic spectrum, different from that of CO_2. The gas sample passes through a chamber crossed by an infra-red beam directed at an infra-red detector in the opposite side. The larger the content of CO_2 in the sample, the lesser is the energy of the beam reaching the detector. Available instruments, measuring CO_2, N_2O and a volatile anaesthetic, are provided with three infra-red beams, at different wavelengths, chosen to coincide with the highest peaks of the infra-red absorption spectrum of each gas.

Most clinical capnographs (sidestream) contain a suction pump pulling a small amount (50–200 ml/min) of gas from the patient's airway via a long sampling tube (Fig. 5), into the analysing cell within the apparatus, thus introducing a delay in the reading (0.1–0.3 seconds) due to the travelling time between the point of sampling and the sensor. Instruments are also

available with a miniaturized sensor placed directly on the breathing system (mainstream), avoiding some problems of the sidestream sampling. This sensor, however, is vulnerable to physical damage and is very expensive.

Clinical case 24

A patient admitted to the intensive care unit, with a provisional diagnosis of an overdose including an opiate drug, has been urgently intubated and placed on a mechanical ventilator following a period of deterioration of efforts to breathe spontaneously. Despite normal ventilator settings for the patient's size and absence of physical signs and history of lung pathology, the readings obtained from the pulse oximeter show a saturation of 81% with a clear, good amplitude pulsation. The capnograph trace shows a slow rise in CO_2 concentration during expiration, never reaching a plateau. There are no leaks or obstructions in the breathing system linking the patient to the ventilator, inspired oxygen concentration is 60% and the chest wall moves with each ventilation cycle.
See comment on page 124.

Oximetry and capnography

- Pulse oximetry and capnography have become indispensable monitoring devices in the settings of anaesthesia and intensive care.
- Both techniques are non-invasive.
- Pulse oximetry indicates oxygenation of arterial blood and capnography indicates adequacy of ventilation.
- Data provided by these instruments is susceptible to artifacts.
- Knowledge of the operating principles of pulse oximetry and capnography is desirable for appropriate interpretation of the readings.

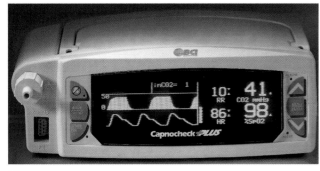

(a)

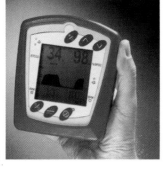

(b)

Fig. 4 **(a)** Monitor showing oximeter and capnograph traces. **(b)** Portable combination pulse oximeter and capnograph.

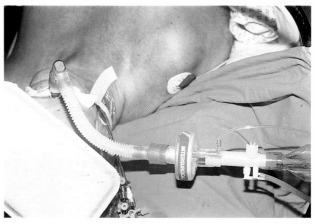

Fig. 5 **Sampling tube of a 'sidestream' capnograph.**

Postoperative recovery

At the end of a surgical procedure, irrespective of whether it was carried out under regional or general anaesthesia, patients can have an unstable cardiovascular system. In addition, those who have had a general anaesthetic may still be unconscious and unable to protect or maintain their airway. Clearly, it would be unacceptable to return such patients directly to a general ward.

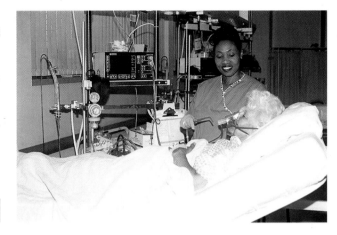

Fig. 1 **One-to-one attention of staff is vital in the recovery room.**

The recovery room

For the post-anaesthetic patient, the recovery room bridges the period leading to the return of consciousness, full return of protective airway reflexes and resumption of spontaneous respiration and cardiovascular stability (depending upon the type of anaesthetic and surgery). In addition to supervising the return of normal physiological function (See 'Core functions', below), recovery room staff ensure that the patient is not bleeding, nauseous or hypothermic, has adequate pain relief and has been prescribed appropriate analgesia and intravenous fluids prior to return to the ward (Table 1). Depending upon local guidelines, and the type and nature of the anaesthesia and surgery, patients will remain in the recovery room for between 30 minutes and 1 hour.

In some situations, particularly after major surgery, some patients may require an extended period of close supervision of the sort provided in the recovery room. This may be because of continuing cardiovascular instability, the need for respiratory support and monitoring, increased risk of bleeding or problems related to an underlying medical condition. These patients may be admitted directly to a high-dependency unit (HDU – sometimes referred to as a progressive care unit, PCU) or to an intensive care unit, until the required degree of physiological stability has been achieved.

The recovery room provides, on a one-to-one basis (Fig. 1), staff skilled in airway management and basic life-support. Recovery staff will closely supervise the post-anaesthetic patient until consciousness has returned. Thereafter, the patient will be regularly monitored until discharge criteria (Table 2) have been satisfied and the patient is able to return to the ward.

Core functions of the recovery room

In many ways, comparison can be made between the situation of the post-anaesthetic patient and that of an individual requiring resuscitation. A direct analogy exists between the principles of recovery room care and those of basic life-support. Hence, on arrival, the post-anaesthetic patient is checked for:

Airway integrity and patency

Unless the patient arrives in the recovery room fully conscious, the anaesthetist will often have left an airway device, such as a Guedel airway, laryngeal mask or endotracheal tube, in place. The recovery room nurse must check that the airway is patent and be ready to suction secretions or vomit.

Breathing

The patient should be breathing spontaneously, and there should be no evidence of airway obstruction. An oxygen mask should be applied and the patient attached to a pulse oximeter to check oxygen saturation. Extending the patient's neck or repositioning the airway may be helpful in treating minor degrees of airway obstruction. If airway obstruction persists, an anaesthetist should be called.

Many anaesthetics involve the use of muscle relaxant drugs and patients may be unable to breathe adequately if these drugs have not been fully reversed. Simple clinical tests such as coughing, head-raising and hand-squeezing may reveal whether there is residual muscle weakness. If residual weakness is suspected, it should be reported to the anaesthetist and treated urgently.

Table 1	**Extended functions and observations of the recovery room.**	
Additional function	**Observation**	**Comment**
Nausea	Patients vomits or complains of nausea	If not already administered, anti-emetic may be needed. Aspirate from nasogastric tube if present
Pain	Pain score high or verbal complaint of pain	Administer prescribed analgesia/start regime after checking previous administration. If shivering, see below
Hypothermia	Patient shivering, complains of cold. Rectal temperature decreased	Apply warm air blower or reflective 'space' blanket. Shivering can occur after GA when normothermic. Shivering increases oxygen requirements
Hyperthermia	Patient may feel hot, may be sweating or have a tachycardia	Measure temperature. May indicate transfusion reaction, sepsis or malignant hyperpyrexia. Summon help
Postoperative drugs	Absent or unused drug chart	Adequate and appropriate analgesia should have been prescribed to avoid delays in administration
Postoperative fluids		Sufficient fluids to cover the first 24 hours postoperatively

Circulation

Pulse and blood pressure should now be checked. Tachycardia and hypotension may mean that the patient is hypovolaemic and requires transfusion.

The patient should remain under one-to-one supervision until consciousness is regained and he or she is able to maintain their airway.

Extended functions of the recovery room

In addition to supervising safe return to consciousness, recovery staff ensure that the patient is not nauseated or in pain, and initiate appropriate treatment where necessary. Postoperative regimes for infusion of analgesic drugs via the epidural, intravenous or subcutaneous routes may be started. The extended functions of the recovery room staff are summarised in Table 1.

Basic requirements

Staffing and equipment

Recovery room staff should be highly skilled in the care of post-anaesthetic patients. They should be able to recognize and initiate basic treatment for all the problems alluded to above, both rapidly and effectively. There should be an effective call system to allow skilled help to be summoned quickly. Staff should undergo regular periods of skills retraining and re-education.

Table 2 **Recovery room discharge criteria**

Parameter	Value	Comment
Level of consciousness	Awake or immediately awakens to command	Patient must have recovered from the anaesthetic and has not been over-sedated by the postoperative analgesia
Airway	No obstruction Can cough effectively and swallow secretions	Patient must be able to maintain and protect airway from secretions and vomit
Breathing	Respiratory rate > 10	Adequate rate and depth of respiration necessary Patient should have oxygen saturations > 95% in room air
Circulation	Mean arterial pressure > 65 mmHg	Patient should have warm, well-perfused peripheries, with no peripheral cyanosis There should be no evidence of bleeding or hypovolaemia Dressings and drains should be checked
Temperature	36.5–37.5°C	Shivering can cause wound pain Wet or soiled linen and bedclothes should be changed
Pain	Little or no discomfort	Patients should be comfortable, able to sleep or rest, but not over-sedated
Nausea	No nausea	See section on nausea and vomiting

In order to fulfil their responsibilities, recovery room staff require full, modern monitoring equipment of the highest standard, piped oxygen supplies and effective suction units. Oxygen masks, airways and other anaesthetic equipment should be readily to hand (see Fig. 2).

Discharge criteria

Before post-anaesthetic patients can safely return to the ward, they should satisfy a number of criteria (Table 2). The criteria listed are suggestions only and may vary between units and in certain clinical circumstances.

> ### Clinical case 25
>
> A 37-year-old female patient has returned to the recovery room following laparoscopic surgery. She has a laryngeal mask airway and her breathing is shallow at a rate of 26 per minute. Despite supplementary oxygen, peripheral saturation is only 94%. Her hands and feet are warm and appear over-perfused, but her tympanic temperature is 35.5°C. She is unresponsive and fine twitching movements are observed in the upper limbs, shoulders and facial muscles.
> *See comment on page 124.*

Fig. 2 **Essential equipment includes oxygen masks, airways and other anaesthetic equipment.**

> ### Postoperative recovery
>
> - The recovery room is a transition point between the operating theatre and the general ward.
> - There is a dedicated nurse for every patient in the recovery room.
> - Vital signs and levels of consciousness are closely monitored.
> - Supplementary oxygen is provided to all patients.
> - Resuscitation equipment is available and staff trained in emergency management are present.
> - Patients must meet certain criteria, including adequate analgesia, before being discharged to the ward.

Practical procedures

Many practical procedures other than the surgery itself are required during the perioperative period, ranging from straightforward to more complex procedures. Adequate training and supervision are essential when learning a new procedure.

Peripheral venous access

Securing intravenous access for administration of fluids, drugs and blood products is essential. Likelihood of maintaining a clean site (see Fig. 1), ease of access, patient comfort, and avoidance of veins crossing joints are important considerations in choosing a site. Topical local anaesthetic preparations such as Amethocaine or EMLA® are useful in needle-phobic patients.

Technique

Choose suitable vein and apply tourniquet proximally. Clean skin with alcohol swab. Infiltrate skin overlying vein with local anaesthetic. Hold skin taut, and insert cannula with needle through skin. (Fig. 2) Advance cannula and needle into vein until flashback obtained. Smoothly advance cannula over needle into vein. Withdraw needle and secure cannula with clean and transparent dressing. Always check patency/position with saline flush before giving drugs or starting infusion.

Central venous access

If it proves impossible to gain peripheral access, central venous cannulation may be necessary (Fig. 3). Central lines are also needed for administration of certain drugs. Central venous pressure monitoring provides a useful guide to intravenous fluid therapy. Attempted insertion of central venous lines carries the risk of significant complications, including pneumothorax, arrhythmias, air embolism, arterial puncture, infection and failure to cannulate the vein. Experienced help and supervision should be sought.

The internal jugular vein can usually be felt or balloted, and pressure may be applied if bleeding occurs. A high approach carries a low risk of pneumothorax. Subclavian vein cannulation carries a greater risk of pneumothorax, and accidental arterial puncture may be difficult to recognize and manage. The femoral vein may be useful, especially if upper body injuries are present, although it is difficult to maintain sterility. The basilic vein may be cannulated with a long line.

This procedure requires a cooperative patient and a full explanation should be given. A trained assistant must be available to help (Table 1). See also page 72.

Insertion of internal jugular line cannula using Seldinger technique

Position patient with neck extended, head-down tilt. Clean skin with alcohol-based antiseptic. Drape area identified. Infiltrate skin and subcutaneously with lignocaine 1%. Flush cannula with saline. Insert needle at midpoint of line adjoining sternal notch and mastoid process, lateral to carotid artery. Advance needle in horizontal plane, towards ipsilateral nipple, aspirating continuously. Once venous blood easily aspirated, remove syringe. Gently feed guide wire through needle, watching ECG. Stop if any resistance. Remove needle and insert dilator over wire. Remove dilator and insert cannula over wire. Remove

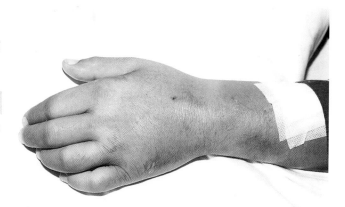

Fig. 1 **One consequence of not maintaining a clean injection site: phlebitis.**

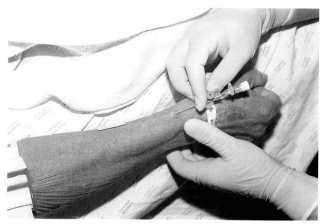

Fig. 2 **Insertion of cannula.** Note proximal tourniquet.

guidewire. Check venous blood can be aspirated from each lumen. Secure and flush with heparinized saline. CXR – rule out pneumothorax and check cannula position.

Care of central venous cannulae

Minimal handling of the line and observance of asepsis when administering drugs and fluids reduce the likelihood of infection. Evidence of local or systemic sepsis for which there is no other identifiable source necessitates line removal (see page 73). Parenteral nutrition and blood products should ideally have a dedicated line. If a vasoactive drug such as dopamine has been infused via the cannula, care must be taken when administering other drugs or fluids as a bolus.

Table 1 **Equipment needed for central line insertion**
■ Tilting bed.
■ ECG monitor.
■ Sterile dressing pack.
■ Sterile gown, gloves and drapes.
■ Alcohol based skin preparation.
■ Lignocaine 1%.
■ Suitable cannula (single or multi lumen).
■ Non-absorbable suture.
■ Sterile transparent dressing.
■ Heparinized saline flush.
■ Pressure monitoring system.
■ CXR facility

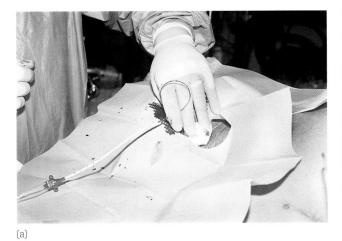 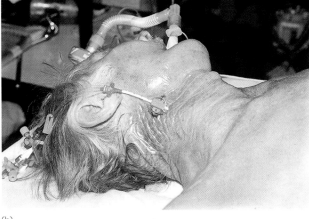

(a) (b)
Fig. 3 **Central venous cannulation. (a)** Insertion of cannula. **(b)** Cannula in situ.

To prevent a bolus of a potent drug, a volume of 10 ml should be aspirated from the line and discarded.

Removal of a central venous line carries the risk of air embolus. Head-down positioning while withdrawing the catheter reduces this risk, and a sterile occlusive dressing should be applied to the puncture site. Bleeding may be a problem on removal, so efforts to correct any coagulopathy are worthwhile.

Arterial blood sampling

Arterial samples may be required to check adequacy of ventilation and severity of metabolic derangement. Possible sites include the radial (ideally non-dominant hand), brachial, dorsalis pedis and femoral arteries. When using the radial site check for collateral flow in the ulnar artery.

Technique
Clean the skin overlying the artery with an alcohol swab, and infiltrate with local anaesthetic. Advance the needle through the skin into the artery proximally at a 30° angle. Aspirate the arterial sample into a heparinized syringe and analyse immediately or store on ice and transfer to the laboratory. Apply firm pressure to the puncture site for 5 minutes to prevent haematoma formation.

Nasogastric tube insertion

Decompression of the stomach is commonly required after abdominal surgery and trauma. Nasogastric tubes may be used for feeding purposes. Orogastric tubes should be used if basal skull fracture is suspected.

Technique
Ensure the patient is in a comfortable sitting position. Estimate the length of tubing required to reach the stomach (usually 35–40 cm). Take a tube and lubricate with lignocaine gel before inserting it gently into the nostril. Advance the tube along the floor of the nose. Once in the nasopharynx, ask the patient to swallow and continue advancing. Check that gastric contents can be aspirated and auscultate over the stomach for a gurgle on injection of air. Secure firmly in place and check the position of the tip of the tube on X-ray.

Bladder catheterization

Open a sterile catheterization pack. Don sterile gloves and clean exposed genital area thoroughly. In male patients it may

be necessary to retract the foreskin. Aim to keep one hand clean throughout the procedure to use for catheter insertion. Insert lignocaine gel into the urethral opening and wait for it to take effect. Remove the tip of the catheter wrapping, and gradually insert the catheter into the urethra directly from the wrapper in order to minimize handling.

In females the urethra is short and the procedure should be straightforward. In males insertion may be tricky, but elevation of the shaft of the penis may help to straighten out the urethra (see Fig. 4). Stop if resistance is felt or the procedure is painful. Once the catheter is inserted fully inflate the balloon with 10 ml sterile water. Stop if this causes pain as the balloon may still be in the urethra. Replace the foreskin if it is retracted.

Urine should flow as soon as the catheter is in the bladder, but sometimes the outlet becomes blocked with gel. Gentle suprapubic pressure, aspiration or flushing should solve the problem.

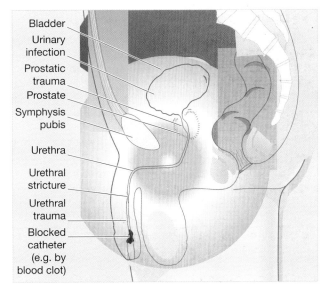

Fig. 4 **Male bladder catheterization route and potential pitfalls.**

Practical procedures
- Always explain procedures to awake patients.
- Maintain aseptic technique.
- Use local anaesthetic/analgesia as required.
- Only carry out procedure for which you have received adequate training
- Seek help if the procedure proves difficult.

Intraoperative complications

When healthy people undergoing minor surgery suffer unexpected injury, this is a tragic and usually preventable outcome. Intraoperative complications are incidents of patient harm occurring during surgical procedures. Such events are frequently preceded by a critical incident, a warning of impending disaster.

Complications may be anaesthetic, surgical or medical in nature, and range in severity from minor injury to debilitation or death. The likelihood of complications increases when patients are medically compromised or surgery is extensive and prolonged. It is imperative to identify those at risk and to endeavour to minimize the risk of complications before they occur. If critical incidents are recognized, complications may be averted and severe adverse outcome may be prevented (Fig. 1).

Critical incidents

A critical incident is an event with the potential to cause harm if allowed to progress. Critical incidents should be preventable by changes in practice, hence the necessity to document and review them (see Table 1). Critical incident coordinators in hospitals ensure that mechanisms are in place for the reporting of incidents and that resources are directed towards the prevention of similar events. The Royal College of Anaesthetists recommends that the severity of outcome of incidents should be scored as follows:

- 0 = No effect
- 1 = Transient abnormality unnoticed by the patient
- 2 = Transient abnormality with full recovery
- 3 = Potentially permanent but not disabling damage
- 4 = Potentially permanent disabling damage
- 5 = Death

Respiratory

Critical incidents and complications involving the respiratory system account for roughly 25% of untoward intraoperative events. The net result of the majority of these is hypoxia, which is life-threatening unless immediately treated.

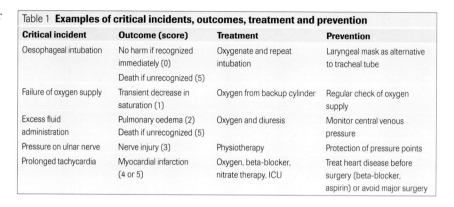

Table 1 Examples of critical incidents, outcomes, treatment and prevention

Critical incident	Outcome (score)	Treatment	Prevention
Oesophageal intubation	No harm if recognized immediately (0) Death if unrecognized (5)	Oxygenate and repeat intubation	Laryngeal mask as alternative to tracheal tube
Failure of oxygen supply	Transient decrease in saturation (1)	Oxygen from backup cylinder	Regular check of oxygen supply
Excess fluid administration	Pulmonary oedema (2) Death if unrecognized (5)	Oxygen and diuresis	Monitor central venous pressure
Pressure on ulnar nerve	Nerve injury (3)	Physiotherapy	Protection of pressure points
Prolonged tachycardia	Myocardial infarction (4 or 5)	Oxygen, beta-blocker, nitrate therapy, ICU	Treat heart disease before surgery (beta-blocker, aspirin) or avoid major surgery

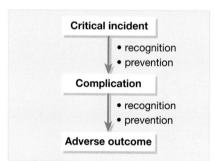

Fig. 1 **Course of a critical incident, and how recognition and prevention can prevent progression to adverse outcome.**

Events amenable to reversal include tracheal tube malposition, laryngospasm, bronchospasm, pneumothorax and oxygen failure. The routine usage of a stethoscope, pulse oximeter, capnograph and oxygen analyser plus careful observation of the patient provide an early warning and may reveal underlying problems.

Cardiovascular

During many operations transient haemodynamic disturbances occur, most of which go unreported, as they are seldom associated with adverse outcomes. Cardiovascular complications are best prevented by identifying those at risk prior to surgery and treating their heart disease, or by opting for a surgical intervention that constitutes less of a physiological infringement. Critical incidents include bradycardia, tachycardia, arrhythmia, hypotension, hypertension and myocardial ischaemia.

Equipment-related

Equipment-related critical incidents should never occur, yet account for a significant proportion of such events. Several simple rules apply when using equipment:

- Never use equipment with which you are unfamiliar.
- Ensure that equipment has been recently serviced.
- Never use equipment for a purpose for which it is not licensed.
- Always check equipment before use (Fig. 2).
- Have emergency back-up equipment available.

If these rules are not followed, there is no defence when equipment-related disaster occurs.

Complications

Complications are the adverse outcomes of critical incidents and are many and varied, depending on the patient's medical history, the skill of staff and the procedure being carried out. Complications range from being transient or unnoticed by the patient to severe causing permanent damage or fatality.

Management

There are 'three ARMs' to the appropriate management of intraoperative complications. A thorough preoperative assessment (A)

Table 2 Examples of intraoperative complications

	Transient (potentially)	Permanent (potentially)
Minor	Sore throat	Nerve damage
	Spinal headache	Chipped teeth
Major	Airway trauma	Death
	Pneumothorax	Brain damage
	Cardiac failure	Stroke
	Cardiac arrest	Eye injury
	Respiratory arrest	Renal failure
	Aspiration pneumonitis	Nerve plexus injury

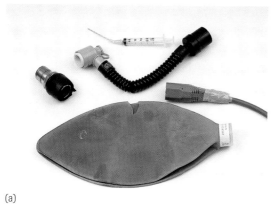

(a)

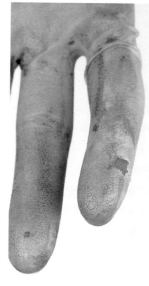

(b)

Fig. 2 **(a) Equipment whose continued usage constitutes a risk. (b) Example of a critical incident: torn glove.** Possible complication: transmission of blood-borne infection.

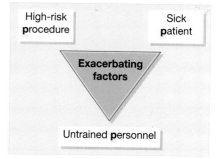

Fig. 3 **Factors exacerbating risk.**

- Possibly preventable with additional resources.
- Probably not preventable.

'A doctor must never conceal from a patient exactly what he did and why.'
Lord Donaldson

allows identification of those at risk. Patients should be warned about the likelihood of complications so that they may make an informed decision about the proposed surgical intervention. When complications do arise, it is crucial that they are recognized (R) so that damage limitation may be attempted. Optimal management (M) of the complication is imperative and this includes honest communication with the patient and counselling.

Documentation and critical incident reporting

The documentation of complications occurring during surgical procedures is vital, both with regards to the future medical management of the patient and possible litigation. Documentation in patient notes provides information, presents a chronological record of events, affords staff protection and ensures accountability.

It is essential that records are comprehensive and accurate with the author, date and time clearly identified, as well as the patient's name and hospital number filled in. Where consent is required, it is important that all common, procedure-specific complications are discussed with the patient and documented. Informed consent may thus be demonstrated.

Clinical Tip
- Poor records = poor defence.
- No records = no defence.

Critical Incident Reporting involves the anonymous declaration of all critical incidents and complications for audit purposes. Incidents are categorized according to their outcome for the patient and their preventability. Critical Incident Reports serve to educate individual health practitioners and departments, and allow risk-management teams to assess the prevalence of various incidents, highlight areas of unsafe practice and recommend changes in practice and protocols.

Critical Incidents do not include all adverse incidents, but rather those events which could have been prevented and which have occurred either due to active failure (human error, these may be errors of omission or commission), or latent failure (inadequate staff training, poor equipment, etc). The prevention of complications is aimed primarily at avoiding those events which are most common in clinical practice and which result in litigation, compensation, and carry the greatest personal cost to the patient.

Preventability scores
- Preventable with current resources.
- Preventable with additional resources.
- Possibly preventable with current resources.

Clinical case 26

Complete a critical incident form to describe the following sequence of events. A senior house officer was administering sedation to a healthy patient for a gastroscope insertion. Oxygen was administered via nasal prongs and the patient was taking 5 breaths/min. The patient started to look a bit blue around the lips, and the pulse oximeter showed a heart rate of 45 beats/min with a peripheral saturation of 85%. It was rapidly ascertained that there was no oxygen flowing through the nasal cannulae. An oxygen cylinder was used to provide oxygen and it was subsequently discovered the oxygen pipeline had disconnected from the wall socket. The patient's oxygen saturation rapidly increased to 99% and the patient suffered no harm.
See comment on page 124.

Intraoperative complications
- Critical incidents are heralds of impending complications.
- Critical incidents are usually preventable with a change in practice.
- The outcome of an incident ranges from no harm to death.
- Accurate documentation at the time of an event is essential.
- Anonymous critical incident reports may prevent recurrence of similar incidents.

Postoperative neurological complications

Postoperative neurological complications constitute rare but devastating events. Some operations carry a particularly high risk. The incidence of confusion in the elderly following orthopaedic surgery approaches 50% and the risk of stroke after carotid endarterectomy is 4%. Neurological complications may be divided into peripheral and central nervous system problems. (Fig. 1)

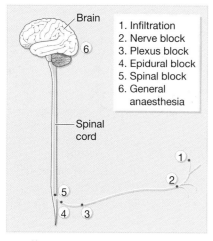

Brain	1. Infiltration
	2. Nerve block
	3. Plexus block
	4. Epidural block
	5. Spinal block
	6. General anaesthesia
Spinal cord	

Fig. 1 **Central and peripheral nervous system.**

Central nervous system complications

Stroke

Both embolic and haemorrhagic stroke may occur during surgery but do not manifest until emergence from anaesthesia. Risk-factors include carotid bruits, history of stroke or transient ischaemic attacks, myocardial infarction, thrombophilia, cardiac surgery and atrial fibrillation. A stroke may be suspected if there is delayed postoperative arousal or loss of function.

Risk may be modified in several ways:

- Maintenance of cerebral perfusion pressure (Fig. 2).
- Tight blood glucose control.
- Adequate oxygen delivery to the brain.
- Cerebral function monitoring.
- Normothermia or mild hypothermia.

Delayed waking following anaesthesia may be indicative of neurological injury. Underlying mechanisms may be decreased cerebral perfusion, hypoxia, increased intracranial pressure or undetected head injury. Metabolic derangement, hypothyroidism, adrenal insufficiency and various drugs have all

been implicated as causes of delayed arousal. Postoperative hypoglycemia should be excluded, especially in diabetics who have received insulin or chlorpropamide before the operation. Patients with sepsis, pancreatitis, pneumonia, uraemia and burns can present with somnolence. Electrolyte abnormalities, especially deranged sodium, depress consciousness. Underlying causes should be identified and treated, bearing in mind that the rapid correction of certain abnormalities, like hyponatraemia, may be dangerous.

Confusion

Postoperative confusion or delirium occurs frequently. Elderly patients following orthopaedic surgery are particularly susceptible. There are several causes for confusion and it is important to identify any correctable mechanisms, for example delirium may be due to pain. Any of the factors causing delayed arousal may underlie confusion.

When patients are excited and agitated on waking, this is termed emergence delirium. This is more common in healthy individuals following painful operations or procedures with high emotional burdens, like amputation. Treatment is with sedatives and analgesia, however, it is imperative to exclude hypoxia. Postoperative cognitive dysfunction is dealt with on page 37.

Convulsions

The most common cause of convulsions in the postoperative period is omission of anticonvulsant therapy. Precipitants of seizures include hypoxia, sodium abnormalities, hypoglycaemia and alcohol withdrawal. Intravenous glucose

and thiamine may be life-saving. Certain surgical procedures carry high risk, especially carotid endarterectomy, cardiac surgery and neurosurgery. Local anaesthetics administered via any route may reach toxic levels and cause seizures. The treatment of fitting involves administration of anticonvulsants, typically benzodiazepines, and the correction of any underlying disorder. Oxygen should always be provided.

Treatment of status epilepticus

- Basic life-support, including oxygen.
- Consider thiamine 100 mg iv or 50 ml 50% glucose iv.
- Lorazepam 4 mg iv or midazolam 10 mg im.
- Phenytoin 15 mg/kg iv over 20 minutes.
- Propofol 2 ml/kg followed by infusion (administered by anaesthetist).

Paraplegia

The mechanism of injury may be direct injury to the spinal cord or ischaemia and infarction. Precautions include the avoidance of low blood pressure and general principles of cerebral protection apply. When a new paraplegia is identified, possible interventions include steroids and continuous aspiration of CSF to decrease intracranial pressure. Urgent neurological assessment is indicated.

Complications of spinal and epidural anaesthesia

Five main neurological complications are associated with spinal and epidural anaesthesia: headache, visual complications, auditory complications, permanent neurological deficits and infection. (Fig. 3)

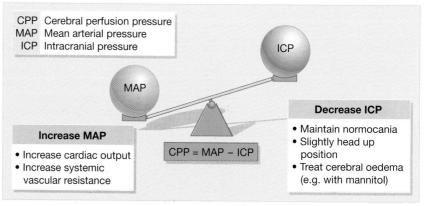

CPP	Cerebral perfusion pressure
MAP	Mean arterial pressure
ICP	Intracranial pressure

Increase MAP
- Increase cardiac output
- Increase systemic vascular resistance

CPP = MAP − ICP

Decrease ICP
- Maintain normocania
- Slightly head up position
- Treat cerebral oedema (e.g. with mannitol)

Fig. 2 **Maintenance of cerebral perfusion pressure.**

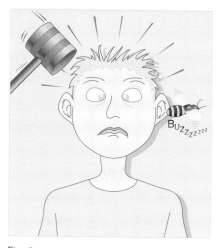

Fig. 3 Neurological complications of spinal and epidural anaesthesia.

Headache

Leakage of CSF from the needle tract causes intracranial hypotension and headache. When an epidural needle breeches the dura, headache is almost invariable. Supine positioning, simple analgesia and generous hydration improve the headache. If the symptoms are refractory, an anaesthetist may perform an epidural blood patch, which usually brings immediate relief.

Visual impairment

The most common visual complications are double vision and blurred vision, both of which are believed to occur following changes in subarachnoid pressure.

Auditory

Tinitus, buzzing and popping are described and are probably due to changes in cochlea pressure.

Neurological deficits

These may be caused by direct trauma or following compression by an epidural haematoma, which must be treated with a decompressive laminectomy within 8–12 hours. Anticoagulated patients may be at higher risk. Deficits produced by direct trauma with the needle are usually permanent and treatment is supportive with physiotherapy and rehabilitation. Regular neurological monitoring is indicated for patients who have had neuraxial (spinal or epidural) blockade. If there is non-resolving paraplegia, incontinence or severe back pain at the needle insertion site, a neurosurgical opinion sought.

Infection

Infection can be introduced into the CSF or epidural space (see Fig. 4). The source of infection may be exogenous from contaminated equipment or drugs, or endogenous from bacteria on the skin of the patient. Meningitis can complicate infection especially if the patient has bacteraemia before the procedure. Prophylaxic antibiotic treatment may prevent meningitis. Other infections include chronic adhesive arachnoiditis and epidural abscess.

Peipheral nerve complications

These may arise following trauma with a needle, stretching or compression of a nerve. Patients at higher risk include diabetics, thin patients and alcoholics. Other risk-factors include the type of surgery, length of the procedure (greater than 6 hours) and the positioning during the operation.

The most frequent peripheral neuropathy is due to abduction of the arm more than 90°. Patients complain of paraesthesia with motor loss generally greater than sensory loss and the upper arm more involved than the hand.

Damage to the common peroneal nerve may result when a patient is lying in the lateral position with the leg resting on the table, and the ulnar nerve is often compressed between the medial elbow joint and the edge of the table or arm board.

These complications are avoided if the patient is placed in natural anatomical positions, arm abduction is restricted and pressure points are cushioned. Rolled towels in the axilla may help. Over 90% of patients make a full recovery within 6 months. Treatment is splinting to prevent deformities and exercise until normal sensation and mobility is regained.

> ## *Clinical case 27*
>
> A 65-year-old woman is on warfarin therapy for atrial fibrillation. Two days ago, a fractured neck of femur was stabilized under epidural anaesthesia. The epidural infusion was discontinued following surgery and warfarin was restarted. She now complains of acute-onset back pain and leg weakness. What should be done?
> *See comment on page 124.*

> ## Postoperative neurological complications
>
> - Reversible causes should always be suspected and treated.
> - Epileptic patients should receive anticonvulsant medications in the perioperative period.
> - Non-resolving paraplegia, incontinence or persistent back pain following spinal or epidural anaesthesia may indicate haematoma and require urgent attention.
> - Protection of pressure points and avoidance of nerve stretching prevents damage to peripheral nerves.

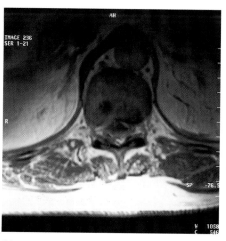

(a)

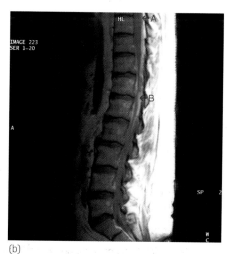

(b)

Fig. 4 (a) Longitudinal and **(b)** transverse MRI scans of the spine (T1-weighted post gadolinium enhancement) showing increased signal (B) obscuring views of the spinal cord (A), in keeping with inflammatory tissue due to infection following epidural catheter placement.

Postoperative cardiovascular complications

Cardiovascular complications occur especially in patients with preoperative risk-factors. As part of the stress response to surgery, there is activation of the sympathetic nervous system. The resultant tachycardia and increased cardiac work, coupled with episodic hypoxaemia, fluid and electrolyte disturbances render the heart vulnerable to ischaemia and arrhythmias.

Blood pressure

Hypotension is sustained systolic blood pressure less than 90 mmHg or mean arterial pressure below 60 mmHg. It is important to identify and treat the underlying causes in order to prevent organ damage or death. The heart, brain, kidney and liver are especially vulnerable during episodes of low blood pressure. Hypoxia and hypovolaemia are life-threatening causes of hypotension, which may occur following surgery and require urgent reversal. Other causes of low blood pressure (Fig. 1) such as sepsis, heart failure, dysrhythmias, anaphylaxis, drug toxicity, epidural analgesia and acid–base abnormalities should be excluded.

Acute hypertension is a sustained elevation of systolic blood pressure above 140 mmHg or diastolic blood pressure above 90 mmHg. This may be associated with cardiac, cerebral and renal morbidity. Before commencing antihypertensive treatment, underlying causes of acute hypertension should be excluded. These include pain, anxiety, hypercapnia, hypoxia, sympathetic activation following surgery, a full bladder, raised intracranial pressure and vasoactive drugs such as dopamine. Unusual causes such as malignant hyperthermia and thyroid storm should be considered. In all instances, supplementary oxygen is indicated.

Arrythmias

Arrhythmias usually occur on a background of pre-existing cardiac disease. Precipitating factors include hypoxia, hypovolaemia, hypercapnia, drug actions, electrolyte abnormalities, acid–base imbalances or a combination of these factors (Fig. 2). Haemodynamic compromise necessitates urgent intervention. A 12-lead electrocardiogram is helpful in establishing a diagnosis. Three simple pieces of information may be gleaned rapidly from the ECG:

- Tachycardia or bradychardia.
- Broad complexes (QRS complex > three small squares) or narrow complexes (see Fig. 3).
- Regular or irregular rhythm.

An appropriate treatment plan may then be devised (see Fig. 4). A heart rate below 40 bpm may be treated with a chronotropic agent or cardiac pacing, the level of intervention being dependent upon the clinical condition of the patient and available expertise. Tachyarrythmias with low blood pressure usually require urgent synchronized cardioversion, for which an anaesthetist should be present to administer sedation. An important exception is a sinus tachycardia, the most common cause of which is hypovolaemia.

When patients are haemodynamically stable, adenosine (6 mg i.v.) is helpful in distinguishing supraventricular from ventricular arrhythmias. Advanced life support courses provide clinicians with the skills and knowledge to cope with many emergency situations. Whenever there is doubt about diagnosis or management, assistance from a cardiologist should be obtained as quickly as possible.

Myocardial ischaemia and infarction

Postoperative myocardial ischaemia is often silent and may not present with the typical signs and symptoms. Chest pain is masked by analgesia, or may be confused with wound pain. Myocardial ischaemia may progress to infarction, whose prognosis is poor when occurring within 48–72 hours of surgery. It is therefore imperative to identify patients at risk, and to maintain vigilance for at least 3 postoperative days.

Following myocardial ischaemia or infarction, priorities include the prevention of hypotension, arrhythmias and heart failure. Pain should be treated aggressively with increments of intravenous morphine. Any ECG changes compared with the preoperative trace may signify an ischaemic event. Cardiac

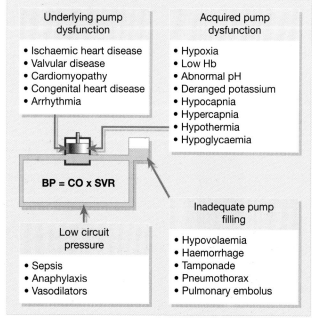

Fig. 1 **Factors affecting blood pressure.**

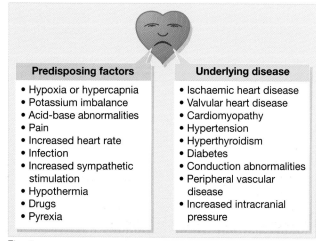

Fig. 2 **Factors predisposing to arrhythmia.**

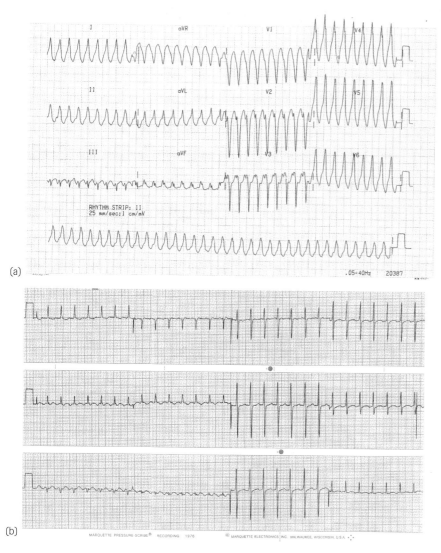

(a)

(b)

Fig. 3 **ECGs showing (a)** broad-complex tachyrrhythmia (ventricular tachycardia – VT) and **(b)** narrow complex tachyrrhythmia (supraventricular tachycardia – SVT).

Troponins (cardiac structural peptides) are sensitive and specific for myocardial injury, except following cardiac surgery.

Beta-blockers, such as atenolol, reduce heart rate, decrease contractility, reduce oxygen demand and have antiarrhythmic properties. Alpha-2-agonists, such as clonidine, may decrease the incidence of perioperative tachycardia and myocardial ischaemia. Glyceryl trinitrate decreases myocardial oxygen demand by reducing preload and increases coronary perfusion pressure (Fig. 5).

Precipitants of postoperative myocardial ischaemia

- H = Hypothermia
- A = Anaemia
- T = Tachycardia
- E = Endotracheal tube
- S = Shivering
- P = Pain
- O = Oxygenation deficiency
- R = REM sleep rebound
- T = Thrombopilia (clotting tendency)

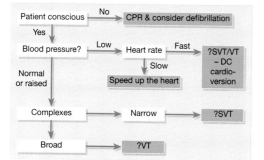

Fig. 4 **Conceptual algorithm for management of arrhythmias.**

Fig. 5 **Factors that decrease the incidence of myocardial ischaemia.**

Postoperative cardiovascular complications

- Cardiac events contribute significantly to postoperative morbidity.
- Hypoxia and hypovolaemia are life-threatening causes of hypotension.
- Monitor oxygenation, heart rate and rhythm, blood pressure, breathing, and temperature.
- Ensure good hydration, adequate analgesia and warmth.
- Provide oxygen to those at risk for at least 3 days following surgery, especially during sleep.
- Antihypertensive and antianginal medications should be restarted following surgery.
- Thrombosis prophylaxis is indicated.

Clinical case 28

A 67-year-old man has undergone femoral popliteal bypass surgery. He has a strong smoking history and is known to have diabetes mellitus, which is well controlled on tablets. He has a low blood pressure following surgery and multiple ventricular ectopic beats on the electrocardiogram trace. What should be done?
See comment on page 124–125.

Postoperative pulmonary complications

The primary functions of the lungs are to transfer oxygen from the atmosphere to the blood and to assist with the removal of carbon dioxide from the body. Postoperative pulmonary complications may impair the lungs' ability to achieve this.

The following are associated with increased risk: preoperative arterial saturation < 90%; age greater than 60 years; obesity; pre-existing lung disease; smoking; upper abdominal and thoracic surgery; prolonged surgery; general anaesthesia.

Airway obstruction

Drowsy patients may be unable to maintain a patent airway. Lying patients on their sides usually prevents the tongue falling back. Oropharyngeal and nasopharyngeal airways allow breathing past the tongue, but may not be tolerated. Airway obstruction is particularly common in those suffering from obstructive sleep apnoea.

Spasm of the vocal cords or laryngospasm is associated with insertion and removal of devices from the upper airway. Such devices include tracheal tubes, laryngeal masks, oropharyngeal airways and suction catheters. Children, asthmatics and those with respiratory tract infections are more susceptible.

Treatment is with humidified oxygen, nebulized epinephrine (adrenaline) and intravenous steroids. Complete obstruction may ensue, necessitating insertion of a tracheal tube.

Bronchospasm is also precipitated by airway manipulation. Asthma, bronchitis, smoking and respiratory tract infections render the airways more irritable. General anaesthesia and intubation are best avoided. Emergency management of bronchospasm is as for severe asthma.

Hypoventilation

The most sensitive marker of hypoventilation is an increase in $PaCO_2$. General anaesthetic drugs are central nervous system depressants and decrease ventilatory drive. Opioid analgesics are particularly potent in this regard. As long as patients are breathing, albeit slowly, they are unlikely to suffer harm as long as they receive supplementary oxygen. Occasionally, patients may require naloxone, but this should only be administered as a last resort as it may precipitate acute pain.

Weakness and impaired diaphragmatic function result in hypoventilation. Residual neuromuscular blockade following non-depolarising muscle relaxants is a treatable cause of weakness. If there is clinical suspicion, a single dose of neostigmine and glycopyrrolate is usually safe. Underlying neuromuscular disease and surgery close to the diaphragm are associated with impaired ventilation.

Atelectasis

Collapse of basal alveoli occurs about 48 hours after surgery. Intrapulmonary shunt leads to a decrease in arterial oxygen saturation. Patients have low-grade pyrexia, tachypnoea and tachycardia in the absence of infection. Chest X-ray occasionally reveals patchy plate-like areas of atelectasis (Fig. 1). Collapse of alveoli renders individuals susceptible to chest infection. Physiotherapy may aid recovery (Fig. 4).

Pneumonia

Retained secretions, atelectasis, pain, abdominal distension and supine position may cause diaghpragmitic splinting. Decreased chest excursions and inability to cough and clear secretions result. Chronic low-grade aspiration of gastric contents allows organisms to gain entry to the lungs (Fig. 2). See page 72.

Aspiration of gastric contents

Aspiration pneumonitis is a chemical inflammation, which may occur following soiling of the lungs with gastric contents. Acute respiratory distress syndrome (ARDS) may result and mortality is high. When aspiration occurs, the priorities are to provide oxygen, to secure and protect the airway and to refer the patient to an intensive care unit.

Pulmonary oedema

The classical clinical features of pulmonary oedema include a distressed,

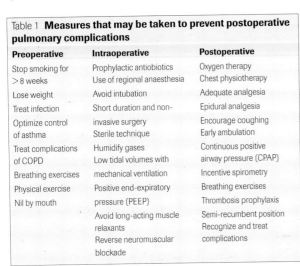

Table 1 **Measures that may be taken to prevent postoperative pulmonary complications**

Preoperative	Intraoperative	Postoperative
Stop smoking for > 8 weeks	Prophylactic antiobiotics	Oxygen therapy
	Use of regional anaesthesia	Chest physiotherapy
Lose weight	Avoid intubation	Adequate analgesia
Treat infection	Short duration and non-invasive surgery	Epidural analgesia
Optimize control of asthma	Sterile technique	Encourage coughing
Treat complications of COPD	Humidify gases	Early ambulation
	Low tidal volumes with mechanical ventilation	Continuous positive airway pressure (CPAP)
Breathing exercises		Incentive spirometry
Physical exercise	Positive end-expiratory pressure (PEEP)	Breathing exercises
Nil by mouth		Thrombosis prophylaxis
	Avoid long-acting muscle relaxants	Semi-recumbent position
	Reverse neuromuscular blockade	Recognize and treat complications

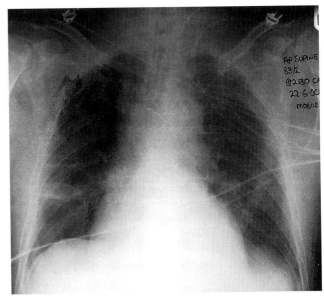

Fig. 1 **Postoperative chest X-ray showing areas of plate atelectasis, seen clearly in the right lower zone.** Notice also the sternal wires, tracheal tube and central venous catheter.

in the second intercostal space in the midclavicular line may be lifesaving.

Pulmonary embolism

Pulmonary embolism is an important cause of death in hospital. There is heightened risk following surgery. All those at risk should receive thrombosis prophylaxis.

Fat embolism syndrome occasionally occurs following major orthopaedic injury involving long bones. Early fixation of fractures may prevent this complication (see case 11 page 27)

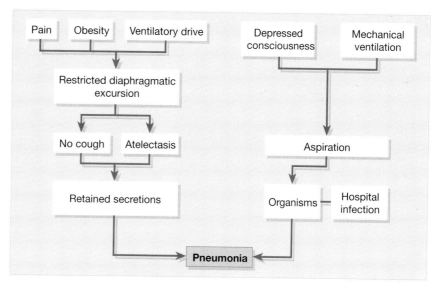

Fig. 2 **Pathogenesis of pneumonia.**

rapid breathing pattern, crackles at the lung bases and the production of pink frothy sputum. Following surgery, it is important to distinguish cardiac from non-cardiac causes. Cardiac failure and fluid overload are treated with oxygen and diuretic therapy.

Negative pressure pulmonary oedema may occur following relief of upper airway obstruction, such as laryngospasm. Treatment is with continuous positive airway pressure (CPAP) or positive pressure ventilation (Fig. 3).

Acute respiratory distress syndrome

The underlying pathology is an increased permeability of the pulmonary capillaries. There is leakage of protein-rich fluid into the lung interstitium and alveoli leading to pulmonary oedema, decreased lung compliance and severe hypoxaemia. ARDS may occur following major trauma, massive blood transfusion, pneumonia, burns, pancreatitis, pulmonary embolism, aspiration, infection in the blood, or following any significant lung injury. This condition is life-threatening and urgent admission to an intensive care unit is indicated.

Pneumothorax

When air enters the pleural cavity and there is compression of a lung, this is termed a pneumothorax. A high index of suspicion is warranted following chest trauma, rib fractures, subclavian central line insertion, performance of brachial plexus block and positive pressure ventilation. A tension pneumothorax may develop if the air leak into the pleural space is sustained. The diagnosis is clinical and intervention may be required before a chest X-ray may be obtained. There is decreased air entry on the affected side with increased resonance to percussion. In severe cases, there is tracheal shift away from the affected side and severe hypotension. Treatment is with an intercostal drain. Emergency insertion of a cannula

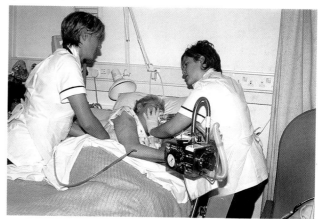

(a)

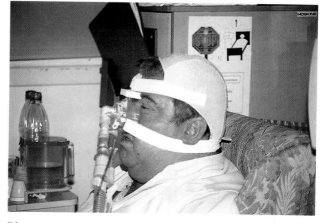

(b)

Fig. 3 **(a) Postoperative respiratory physiotherapy. (b) Continuous positive airway pressure ventilation.**

Postoperative pulmonary complications

- Upper airway obstruction should be distinguished from bronchospasm.
- Pneumothorax and residual neuromuscular blockade are easily reversible.
- Chest X-ray and an arterial blood gas, coupled with history and examination, allow discrimination among the various pulmonary complications.
- Advice from a respiratory physician or an intensivist should be sought early.
- Supplementary oxygen is an immediate priority.

Clinical case 29

A 25-year-old professional football player had emergency appendix surgery. In the ward, he has difficulty breathing, his peripheral saturation is 87% and he is coughing up pink frothy sputum. How should this patient be managed?
See comment on page 125.

Postoperative nausea and vomiting

Nausea is the uncomfortable sensation of an impending episode of vomiting. It is often associated with salivation, swallowing, pallor and tachycardia. Postoperative nausea and vomiting (PONV) is the most common complication necessitating admission following day-surgery. It occurs in 9–15% of all patients and is frequently described as the most unpleasant experience of surgery and anaesthesia. Therefore, identifying those at risk and trying to minimize the incidence is extremely important.

Table 1 Risk factors for and precipitants of PONV

Patient factors	Previous PONV, motion-sickness, obesity, young women and children, perimenstrual women, pregnant women, non-smokers, anxiety
Anaesthetic factors	Hypoxaemia, dehydration hypotension, drugs (etomidate, nitrous oxide, inhalational anaesthesia, opioids, neostigmine), airway instrumentation, gastric insufflation, pain, patient not fasted
Surgical factors	Laprascopic surgery, abdominal surgery, gynaecological surgery, ear, nose and throat surgery, ophthalmologic surgery, knee arthroscopies, long surgery
Co-existing diseases	Migraine (aura), renal failure, delayed gastric emptying Increased intracranial pressure, infection, ileus, diabetes mellitus, epilepsy, myocardial infarction
Other	Gastric irritants, including blood, excessive movement Drugs (opioids, cytotoxics, digoxin, sinemet), nasogastric tube, abdominal distension, hypoglycaemia

Pathophysiology

Nausea and vomiting are activated via afferent pathways, which converge on integrating centres in the central nervous system, which then transmit signals via effector pathways (see Fig. 1). Most sensory pathways can trigger nausea (see Table 1). An unpleasant sight, smell, taste, sensation, sound or even emotion, may act on the limbic cortex, which in turn may communicate with the vomiting centre (VC).

The VC, which resides in the reticular formation of the medulla at the level of the olivary nuclei, also receives inputs from nociceptive (pain) pathways, vestibular apparatus (motion and vertigo), the chemoreceptor trigger zone (CTZ) and the vagus nerve. Acetylcholine and histamine are neurotransmittors which act as agonists at the VC.

The CTZ is circumventricular in the area postrema and lies outside the blood–brain barrier (BBB). Its activation is thus not dependent on substances crossing the BBB. Dopamine, serotonin and various drugs and toxins activate the CTZ. Serotonin also acts via peripheral (5HT3) receptors. Efferent stimuli travel via the vagus nerve to the oesophagus, diaphragm and striated abdominal muscles resulting in closure of the glottis, reverse peristalsis and the forceful expulsion of gastric contents through the mouth.

Prevention and treatment

Various approaches have been attempted to decrease the incidence of PONV. Firstly, those at risk must be identified. Non-pharmacological methods are useful and include avoidance of hypotension and dehydration, hypnosis, acupuncture or acupressure and minimization of patient head movement. Acupressure bands on the P6 meridian or Neiguan pressure point (three finger breadths proximal to the palmer crease) applied before induction of anaesthesia and continued for 6 hours postoperatively has been suggested as prophylaxis against PONV (Fig. 2). There are randomized trials suggesting some efficacy.

Avoidance of pro-emetic drugs, especially opioids, is advocated. However, pain is also a powerful pro-emetic stimulus and unpleasant in its own right. Analgesics other than opioids may achieve adequate analgesia.

Recently, compelling evidence has emerged that, for abdominal surgery (but possibly other operations as well), 80% oxygen given during surgery and for 6 hours postoperatively significantly decreases the incidence of PONV (Fig. 3). This is a safe and cheap intervention, which may also decrease other morbidity, like infection (page 49).

Pharmacological intervention

Before rushing in with pharmacological treatment of PONV, it is important to exclude life-threatening underlying causes, like hypoxia, hypoglycaemia, hypotension and dehydration.

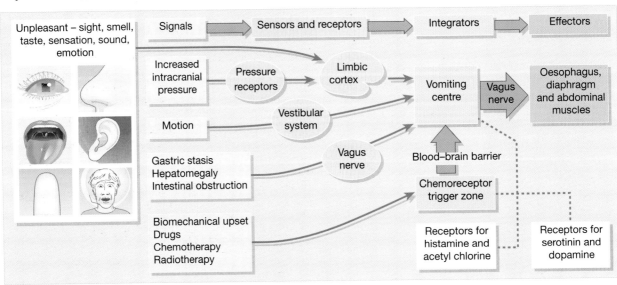

Fig. 1 **Diagramatic representation of the pathophysiology of PONV.**

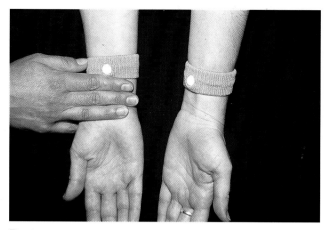

Fig. 2 **Acupressure bands on the P6 meridian or Neiguan pressure point.**

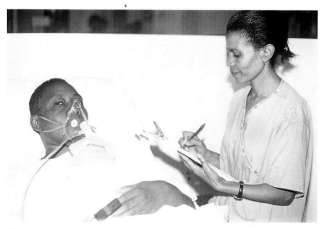

Fig. 3 **Patient receiving high-concentration oxygen following surgery.**

Ginger root, 0.5 mg powdered in a capsule, has been advocated as a natural remedy for nausea. Pharmacological prophylaxis and treatment is usually with an antidopaminergic, an anticholinergic or an antihistaminergic drug (Table 2). If a drug is not effective, it is unlikely that another drug from the same class will provide relief. It is surprising that metaclopromide (10 mg iv) is one of the most commonly used anti-emetic agents, as current data suggest that at this dosage, it has limited efficacy in the treatment of nausea. Nabilone is a synthetic cannabinoid with anti-emetic properties reportedly superior to prochlorperazine. Side-effects including dysphoria and hallucinations are common.

The best approach to the treatment of PONV may be a stepwise or multimodal approach. This entails starting with one agent and then adding drugs with different mechanisms of action until there is some relief. Specific antagonists at serotonergic 5HT3 receptors may be successful where other drugs have failed. There are also fewer side-effects associated with these agents; in particular they do not cause drowsiness. The major downside to 5HT3 blockers is cost. Rapid intravenous administration of the 5HT3 antagonist ondansetron may cause arrhythmias.

Consequences of PONV

Besides being extremely unpleasant, there are other consequences associated with refractory nausea and vomiting. The inability to take anything orally prevents the introduction of feeding and prohibits oral medication. Dehydration and metabolic alkalosis, through loss of gastric secretions, are dangerous complications. The forceful muscle contraction involved in vomiting may cause wound dehiscence. Sympathetic stimulation, in particular tachycardia, may precipitate myocardial ischaemia.

Clinical case 30

Following a hysterectomy during which blood loss was about 1500 ml, a 45-year-old previously healthy woman complains of severe nausea. She received droperidol as prophylaxis against nausea. Blood pressure is 100/50 and heart rate is 120 bpm. What should be done for her?
See comment on page 125.

Postoperative nausea and vomiting

- PONV is a frequent complication of surgery and anaesthesia.
- PONV is the most common cause of unanticipated hospital admission following day-surgical procedures.
- High-concentration oxygen is a cheap, safe and effective means of reducing the incidence of PONV.
- Life-threatening causes of PONV, including hypoxia, hypotension and hypoglycaemia, should be excluded.
- Droperidol 0.25–0.5 mg iv provides cost-effective prophylaxis.
- Multi-modal therapy may be most effective for treatment.
- There are dangerous complications of PONV, in particular metabolic alkalosis and dehydration.

Drug class	Drug and dosage (adult)	Mechanism of action
Anticholinergics	Hyoscine 2–4 mg im	Central anticholinergic action
Antihistamines	Cyclizine 50 mg iv/im	Central antihistaminergic
	Promethazine 100 mg iv	
Butyrophenones	Droperidol 0.5–1 mg iv	Central antidopaminergic
Phenothiazines	Prochlorperazine 12.5 mg im	Central antidopaminergic
5HT₃ antagonists	Ondansetron 4–8 mg iv	Central and peripheral anti-serotonergic
	Granisetron 1 mg iv	
Steroids	Dexamethasone 4 mg iv	? intracranial pressure
GABA agonists	Propofol 10–20 mg iv	? cerebral cortex

Table 2 **Drugs for the treatment of PONV**

?; exact mechanisms of the drugs in treating nausea are unclear.

Postoperative bleeding

Surgery is invariably associated with some degree of bleeding. Certain procedures, such as major arterial surgery and those procedures involving highly vascular tissue (liver, spleen), constitute a high risk for postoperative bleeding. When patients bleed following surgery, a challenge facing the doctor is to distinguish between inadequate surgical haemostasis and a bleeding diathesis. Appropriate early intervention may prevent escalation of the problem.

Haemostasis

Adequate haemostasis depends on interaction among functioning platelets, clotting factors and a surface on which the clot can anchor. Disruption of a vessel wall sets in motion a series of events. Localized vasoconstriction (Fig. 1) decreases blood flow and exposure of underlying collagen, along with other platelet activators, stimulates platelet aggregation into a loosely-formed plug. Simultaneous activation of coagulation by tissue factor results in the production of fibrin, which stabilizes the clot over the breeched vessel. Fibrinolysis is one of the mechanisms preventing inappropriate clot extension, but hyper-fibrinolysis may prevent adequate primary haemostasis.

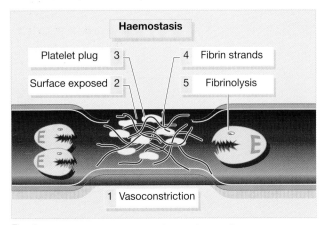

Fig. 1 **Adequate haemostasis relies on interaction among functioning platelets, clotting factors and a surface on which the clot can anchor** (see text).

Bleeding tendencies

Patients with hereditary bleeding tendencies and those taking anticoagulant medications (see pages 16), should be identified preoperatively, and a management plan should be formulated in consultation with a haematologist. The risk of bleeding is also increased in the presence of liver and renal dysfunction. Even those with normal clotting mechanisms at the outset may acquire a coagulapathy during surgery. The following are associated with impaired haemostasis.

- Hypothermia. During general anaesthesia there is a loss of normal thermoregulatory mechanisms and some degree of hypothermia is an almost inevitable consequence. This is aggravated by the transfusion of cold fluids and the cold operating theatre. Hypothermia adversely affects all three major components of haemostasis.

- Hypertension increases blood loss from surgical incisions and impairs the ability of blood to clot.
- Heparin is frequently administered during vascular and cardiac surgery. Heparin inhibits clotting by potentiating the action of antithrombin and may also cause platelet clumping and dysfunction.
- Protamine may be administered to reverse heparin, but excess protamine may itself inhibit coagulation and platelet function.
- Disseminated intravascular coagulation (DIC) may occur secondary to widespread tissue damage and surgery with its attendant bleeding diathesis.
- A dilutional coagulopathy may develop following massive blood loss (two to three times the blood volume). Transfused red cells do not contain platelets or clotting factors.
- Cardiopulmonary bypass. There are multiple factors contributing to a bleeding diathesis following cardiopulmonary bypass. Exposure to the bypass circuit results in consumption of platelets and clotting factors, as well as activation of fibrinolysis. Heparin is given to prevent clotting of the bypass circuit and protamine is administered to reverse heparinization. Inappropriate dosing with either drug may precipitate bleeding. In addition, hypothermia is extremely common following open cardiac surgery.

Preventing bleeding

A detailed history and examination may reveal patients at risk for bleeding and where possible surgery should be avoided or less extensive surgery embarked upon. The importance of keeping patients warm during and after surgery cannot be stressed enough. Using warm intravenous fluids, increasing environmental temperature, employing warm air convection devices and providing adequate insulation may achieve this.

When there is suspicion that a patient has a bleeding diathesis, advice from a haematologist should be sought early. If there is any suspicion that the underlying cause of bleeding is surgical, patients should be returned to the operating theatre for exploration as soon as possible, as ongoing bleeding will lead to the development of a coagulopathy and increase the need for transfusion. Antifibrinolytic drugs, such as aprotinin, tranexamic acid and epsilon-aminocaproic acid reduce blood loss, but may be associated with increased risk of thrombosis, expert advice should be sought.

Diagnosis

Differentiating between a medical and surgical cause of bleeding has important therapeutic implications. A bleeding diathesis usually manifests as generalized ooze rather than bleeding from a specific site. The priority is to exclude readily reversible causes, such as hypothermia and heparin effect.

Laboratory tests

Most haematology laboratories provide a fairly rapid coagulation profile (INR, APTT and fibrinogen levels) as well as a full blood count. A prolonged APTT ($>$ 1.5 times normal) with a normal INR is suggestive of heparin effect. If the INR is $>$ 1.5 with a normal APTT, warfarin effect, undiagnosed haemophilia and vitamin K deficiency are possible diagnoses. A prolongation of both INR and APTT may suggest generalized clotting factor deficiency. Thrombocytopenia may underlie bleeding when the platelet count is below $50 \times 10^9/L$. The problems with haematology laboratory diagnoses are as follows:

- There is a delay before results are available.
- No information is provided about platelet function.
- Fibrinolysis is not detected in standard tests.
- Effects of anticoagulant medications, other than warfarin and heparin, are undetected.

Near-patient haemostatic assessment

Diagnosis of problems underpinning a bleeding diathesis at the bedside allows rapid and targeted intervention (Fig. 2). The activated clotting time (ACT) has been available for many years to assess adequacy of heparin effect, especially during cardiac surgery. A major weakness with the ACT is that it is insensitive to low plasma heparin concentrations (< 3 units/ml), which are nonetheless sufficient to increase bleeding. Bedside INR, APTT and fibrinogen tests are available and may provide valuable information.

Assessment of platelet function is recognized as a priority and machines such as the PFA-100® platelet function analyser and HemoSTATUS® are undergoing clinical evaluation. The

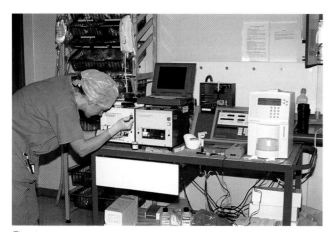

Fig. 2 **Photograph showing the use of near-patient haemostatic assessment devices.**

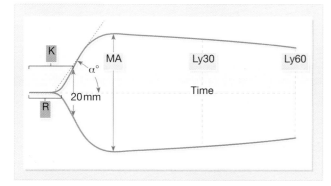

Fig. 3 **A TEG trace.** R and K represent times to clot formation, alpha angle depicts rate of clot extension and MA is reflective of clot strength. Ly30 and Ly60 are indices of clot breakdown or lysis.

thromboelastograph (TEG)®, which was introduced in 1948, has enjoyed a resurgence in recent years. The TEG provides a global view of haemostasis, delivering information about time to clot formation, clot strength (reflecting platelet fibrinogen interaction) and fibrinolysis (see Fig. 3). While there is controversy surrounding the usefulness of the TEG, several trials have demonstrated that the information provided decreases unnecessary blood product transfusion and guides therapeutic intervention.

Management of bleeding

The definitive treatment for surgical bleeding is suture material. A bleeding diathesis should be excluded as rapidly as possible. It is important to treat hypothermia and hypertension quickly and effectively. Where bleeding is peripheral, simple interventions such as elevation and pressure may be sufficient to stem blood loss.

The APTT and machines such as the TEG® and the Hepcon Heparin Management System® provide a sensitive indication of residual heparin effect, which may be reversed with protamine. Empirical administration of protamine may worsen bleeding. An antifibrinolytic medication, such as tranexamic acid 15 mg/kg IV, may be beneficial. Desmopressin (DDAVP 0.3 μmg/kg iv) transiently increases factor VIII and von Willebrand levels, and is associated with a temporary improvement in platelet function. Pooled platelets are indicated when there is diffuse bleeding in the presence of thrombocytopenia (platelet count $< 50 \times 10^9/L$) or suspected platelet dysfunction. Fresh frozen plasma is only appropriate when there is a documented coagulopathy with no readily reversible cause, like heparin, and cryoprecipitate is suggested for hypofibrinogenaemia.

> ### Clinical case 31
> A patient has had routine coronary bypass surgery and 6 hours following surgery has been extubated and transferred to the high-dependency area of the cardiac surgery ward. Chest drains reveal ongoing blood loss exceeding 100 ml/hour. What steps should be taken in managing this problem?
> *See comment on page 125.*

> ### Postoperative bleeding
>
> - It is crucial to distinguish between surgical bleeding and a bleeding diathesis.
> - Surgical exploration should be undertaken sooner rather than later.
> - Hypothermia and hypertension worsen blood loss.
> - Platelet dysfunction and hyperfibrinolysis contribute to postoperative bleeding.
> - Antifibrinolytic drugs and DDAVP may decrease bleeding.
> - Near-patient haemostatic assessment provides information rapidly and allows targeted intervention.
> - Fresh frozen plasma is seldom indicated.

Perioperative infection

Perioperative infections are generally hospital-acquired infections (HAI). Approximately 10% of hospital in-patients develop HAI (Fig. 1), and 1–4% of patients will die of their infection. A third of HAIs may be preventable with infection control and antibiotic policies.

Surgical wards contain patients at high risk of acquisition of HAI. Patients may be elderly and have chronic disorders like diabetes mellitus and vascular disease. Urinary catheters, immobility, intravenous drips, surgical wounds and antibiotic use are risks for the development of HAI.

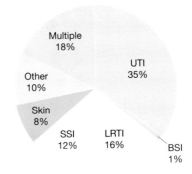

Fig. 1 **Hospital-acquired infections** (LRTI = lower respiratory infection, UTI = urinary tract infection, SSI = surgical site infection, BSI = bloodstream infection).

Surgical site infection

Surgical site infection (SSI) is divided into superficial (involving skin and subcutaneous tissues), deep (fascial and muscle layers) and organ or tissue spaces (any area opened, manipulated during surgery).

Staphylococcus aureus, including MRSA is the predominant cause. Other causative organisms are coagulase negative Staphylococci, Coliforms and *Clostridium perfringens*.

Organ or tissue space infection after gastrointestinal surgery presents as peritonitis or intra-abdominal abscess. Common causative organisms are coliforms, *Pseudomonas aeruginosa*, Candida *spp.* and *Bacteroides fragilis*. Investigations should include a septic screen (see below) and abdominopelvic ultrasound.

Cefuroxime and metronidazole would be appropriate antibiotic therapy for SSI, while awaiting culture results.

Septic screen (first-line investigations)

Blood cultures, FBC, CRP and ESR, MSU, aspiration of pus (sample of pus in sterile jar preferred to swab), CXR

Hospital-acquired pneumonia

Pneumonia should be suspected in the following circumstances: fever > 38°C, leucocytosis, deterioration in gas exchange, radiographic appearance of new infiltrates (Fig. 2) or purulent respiratory secretions

Organisms responsible for hospital acquired pneumonia include *Pseudomonas aeruginosa* (30%), *Staphylococcus aureus*, including MRSA (30%) and coliforms such as *Klebsiella pneumoniae*, *Esherichia coli* and *Enterobacter* spp. (30%).

Suitable empirical therapy for hospital-acquired pneumonia is ceftazidime or pipericillin/tazobactam. Oxygen therapy is usually required.

Urinary catheter-associated infection

Urinary catheterization is the most common risk-factor for urinary sepsis. Following catheterization, 50% of patients are infected at 15 days and 100% after 1 month (Fig. 3). Causative organisms are *E coli*, *Klebsiella spp.*, *Proteus spp.*, *Pseudomonas aeruginosa*, Candida spp., and *Enterococci*.

Suitable oral antibiotics are trimethoprim, nitrofurantoin and coamoxiclav. Ciprofloxacin should be reserved for resistant cases. Intravenous cefuroxime (with gentamicin) can be given to unwell, septic patients with suspected UTI.

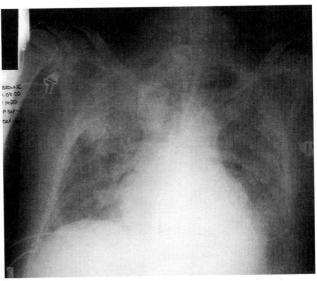

Fig. 2 **Chest X-ray showing widespread consolidation in keeping with nosocomial pneumonia.**

If a urinary catheter is present, it should be removed or replaced if considered vital. An abdominopelvic ultrasound may exclude hydronephrosis and urinary obstruction. Free drainage of urine is essential if the urinary tract is infected. Catheters must be inserted with strict asepsis (see Fig. 3).

Bloodstream infection (BSI)

Infected central and peripheral intravenous catheters are responsible for 50% of cases of BSI. Other causes of BSI are pneumonia, surgical site infection and urinary infection. Infected peripheral lines may be tender, with redness, pus and ascending thrombophlebitis.

Infected central catheters may not be associated with local sepsis at the insertion site. Episodic fever with bacteraemia is common. Causative organisms include coagulase negative *Staphylococci* and *S. aureus* including MRSA. Other culprits include *E coli*, *Pseudomonas* spp. and *Enterococci*.

If line-related infection is suspected, then prompt removal of the line is advised. Empirical therapy with flucloxacillin, or vancomycin if MRSA is prevalent, should be instituted.

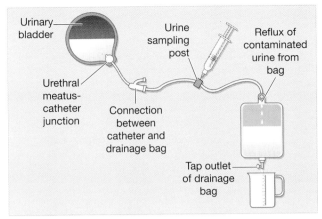

Urinary bladder
Urine sampling post
Reflux of contaminated urine from bag
Urethral meatus-catheter junction
Connection between catheter and drainage bag
Tap outlet of drainage bag

Fig. 3 Points of entry for bacteria in a closed urinary catheter system (reproduced with kind permission from Damani NN. Manual of Infection Control Procedures. Greenwich Medical Media Ltd, 1998).

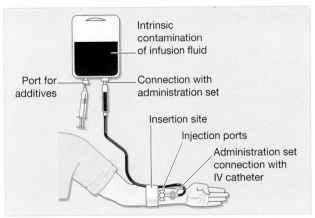

Intrinsic contamination of infusion fluid
Port for additives
Connection with administration set
Insertion site
Injection ports
Administration set connection with IV catheter

Fig. 4 Points of access for bacteria through an intravenous infusion line (reproduced with kind permission from Damani NN. Manual of Infection Control Procedures. Greenwich Medical Media Ltd, 1998).

Intravenous lines, including peripheral lines, should be inserted with strict attention to asepsis. (Fig. 4).

MRSA

Methicillin-resistant *Staphylococcus aureus*, MRSA, is a global problem. It is transmitted between patients, usually on healthcare workers' hands. Strict infection control can curtail its spread, hand hygiene is critical (Fig. 6). Vancomycin, or the related agent, teicoplanin, must be included in the empirical antibiotic regimen of any MRSA-positive patient with suspected infection or for antibiotic prophylaxis. Theatre staff should be made aware of one patient's MRSA status.

Case report – *Clostridium difficile*-associated diarrhoea (CDAD)

A 75-year-old woman developed wound infection following total abdominal hysterectomy. She was started on cefuroxime. After 5 days of treatment, she developed fever (38.8°C), bloody diarrhoea and abdominal cramps. Sigmoidoscopy revealed colitis. *Clostridium difficile*-associated diarrhoea was diagnosed and she was given oral metronidazole. *C. difficile* toxin was subsequently identified in stool.

Since 1992 the reported incidence of *C difficile* infection has increased nine-fold. The aetiology of this disease remains obscure. Reduced colonization resistance of the colon, allowing colonization by *C. difficile* appears to be a key factor. Antibiotic use is the most important risk-factor. The elderly are very susceptible. *C difficile* is associated with a spectrum of clinical presentations from asymptomatic carriage to fulminant pseudomembranous colitis.

Therapy is given according to severity. Oral metronidazole and rehydration is indicated when diarrhoea is persistent and fever present. Metronidazole can be administered intravenously if oral therapy is not possible. Oral vancomycin is second-line therapy.

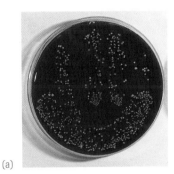

(a)

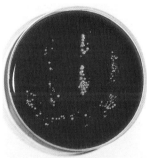

(b)

Clinical case 32

A 39-year-old woman has had a mastectomy for metastatic breast carcinoma and a tunneled central line was inserted for chemotherapy. She is admitted to the ward with nausea, vomiting and dehydration. Intravenous rehydration is commenced through the central line. One hour after the infusion, she becomes pale and sweaty and has a prolonged rigor. Her pulse is 120 bpm, blood pressure drops to 80/40 and her temperature rises to 39°C. What should be done?
See comment on page 125.

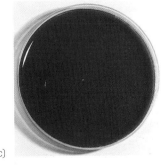

(c)

Fig. 5 Hand impressions with colonies of organisms on blood agar illustrating the effectiveness of hand washing. (a) No hand washing. **(b)** Washing with soap and water. **(c)** Use of alcohol hand rub.

Perioperative infection

■ One in ten patients develop hospital-acquired infection.

■ Common postoperative infections are urinary tract infection, pneumonia, surgical site infection and bloodstream infection.

■ Aseptic technique should be of a high standard when performing urinary catheterization or insertion of an intravenous line.

■ Frequent hand washing is the most effective way of preventing transmission of hospital 'super bugs' like MRSA.

Allergic reactions

Allergic reactions occur frequently in the hospital setting where patients are exposed to a myriad high-risk substances, ranging from antibiotics and latex-containing compounds to intravenous contrast media and blood products. Patients in the perioperative period are particularly vulnerable.

Key terms

- *Anaphylaxis* – a profound, potentially life-threatening, immune-mediated reaction on re-exposure to an allergen.
- *Anaphylactoid reaction* – a profound, potentially life-threatening reaction similar in many respects to anaphylaxis, but not requiring prior exposure to the trigger.
- *Allergen* – a foreign substance (antigen), which may induce an anaphylactic reaction.
- *Immunoglobin or antibody* – a protein produced by the immune system, which can recognize and bind to foreign antigens.
- *Mediators* – chemicals whose release produces the signs and symptoms of anaphylactic and anaphylactoid reactions.
- *Idiosynchratic* reaction – an abnormal susceptibility to a drug or substance peculiar to an individual.

Definition

An allergic reaction takes place when there is an exaggerated response to foreign substances. Food, insect venom, pollen, antibiotics and animal hair frequently precipitate allergic reactions. Severe allergy or anaphylaxis occurs when exposure to an allergen primes the immune system such that subsequent exposure results in an inappropriate hypersensitive immune response, which may be fatal.

Pathology

When an individual is sensitized to an antigen, there is a production of immunoglobin E (IgE) antibodies (Fig. 1). If there is repeat exposure to the same compound, it is recognized by the IgE antibodies. Antibody–allergen complexes bind to mast cells or basophils, inducing degranulation and mediator release.

These released chemicals can have both local and widespread actions. Typically, there are cardiovascular, pulmonary and cutaneous manifestations. Relaxation of smooth muscle in the blood vessels coupled with contraction of smooth muscle in the respiratory tract occurs. If severe, there is a fall in blood pressure and breathing difficulties resembling an acute asthma attack. The

rapid systemic release of large quantities of mediators causes capillary leakage and mucosal oedema, which may result in distributive shock.

This pathological process may also be initiated without prior exposure to a substance. An anaphylactoid reaction occurs when a triggering agent activates the complement cascade or acts directly on mast cells or basophils, thereby precipitating mediator release.

People often describe any problem they may have had with a drug as an allergy. However, it is important to emphasize that a minority of adverse drug reactions are allergic in nature. Far more common are side-effects, toxicity and idiosyncratic reactions.

Risk in hospitalized patients

In the perioperative period, doctors and nurses inject a variety of substances directly into the bloodstream, bypassing the normal defence mechanisms and rapidly achieving high plasma concentrations. This increases the likelihood of allergic-type reactions. Hospitalized patients are exposed to numerous drugs, intravenous fluids, blood components, surgical dressings, and latex-containing substances (Fig. 2). Patients who are anaesthetized, heavily sedated, confused or receiving opioid analgesia are particularly vulnerable, as they may be unable to express the early symptoms of an allergic reaction.

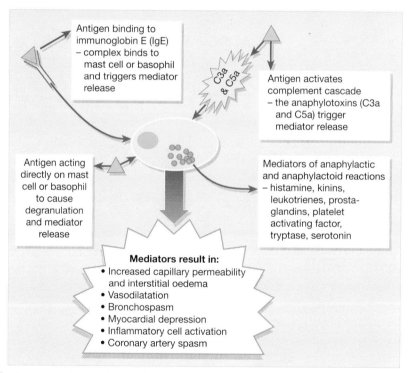

Fig. 1   **Diagram illustrating mechanisms of allergic-type reactions.**

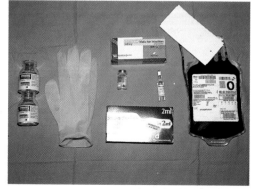

Fig. 2   **Photograph of high-risk substances in the hospital setting** (CLAMP = contrast medium, latex, antibiotics, muscle relaxants, blood products).

Intraoperative allergic reactions are estimated to occur at a rate between 1 in 5000 and 1 in 25 000 and carry a mortality of 3–5%.

The following are associated with a high incidence of allergic-type reactions: Intravenous contrast media; antibiotics, especially penicillin; intravenous anaesthetic agents, especially muscle relaxants; latex-containing products; blood and blood products.

Latex allergy

Latex allergy is a hypersensitivity to the plant proteins in natural rubber (see Fig. 3). Latex sensitivity has prevalence of 1–6% in the general population, and among health workers it is 8–17%. Those who have had significant exposure to latex in early life, like repeated catheterization or multiple surgical procedures, are at particularly high risk. Latex gloves are often implicated as precipitants of allergy and their powder is a source of airborne allergens.

Latex rubber anaphylaxis may develop more slowly (30 minutes or longer from the time of exposure) if the allergen has to be absorbed through the skin or mucosa.

Prevention

There are several important steps that should be taken to avoid allergic reactions:

- Ask patients specifically about their allergies, including latex.
- Enquire about atopy and asthma.
- Look in the patient's notes and check for Medic Alert bracelet.
- Communicate:
  - Document allergies in notes.
  - Write on patient's wristband.
  - Tell other staff members who are involved with the patient.
- Minimize patient exposure to high-risk substances.
- Patients considered to be at risk should not receive drugs which are known to induce histamine release.

Diagnosis of allergy

History Patients with any history of allergy, atopy or asthma are more prone to allergic reactions. Previous exposure to an allergen is important and if past repeated exposure has been uneventful, allergy is unlikely.

Examination Whenever unexplained cardiovascular collapse, bronchospasm, or skin rash occurs, the diagnosis of allergy should be considered. This is particularly so if such an event occurs shortly after exposure to a known allergen. Allergy is a clinical diagnosis and represents a life-threatening medical emergency.

Laboratory Tryptase is released from mast cells and basophils, lasts for up to 4 hours in the blood and may even help in making a post mortem diagnosis. As mast cell tryptase is only increased transiently, blood should be taken when it peaks about 1 hour after the onset of the reaction.

Diagnostic testing Patients who have survived a suspected allergic reaction should have skin testing or serologic tests to confirm sensitivity to the allergen.

Treatment

Epinephrine (adrenaline) should be administered urgently as it treats hypotension, promotes bronchodilation, and inhibits mediator release. The safest method of administering adrenaline may be via an intramuscular injection of 0.5 mg. This avoids the danger of precipitous hypertension with intravenous adrenaline and prevents delays in obtaining intravenous access.

Extensive intravascular volume replacement is usually needed to restore cardiac output in distributive shock. Emergency resuscitation, including chest compressions and advanced airway management, may be necessary in severe cases of allergy.

The allergy treatment A-list

- Cease Administration of drug and call for help.
- Airway – maintain and give 100% oxygen.
- Adrenaline (epinephrine) – 0.5 mg imi or 10–100 µmg ivi.
- Administer fluids – 2–4 litres fast as a temporizing measure to maintain cardiac output.
- β-2-Agonist (nebulized or ivi) and oxygen for bronchospasm.
- Adrenocorticosteroid – hydrocortisone 200 mg ivi or imi.
- Antihistamine – chlorpheniramine 10 mg ivi or imi.
- Adrenaline (epinephrine) or noradrenaline (norepinephrine) infusion.
- Arterial blood gas – treat Acidosis with bicarbonate 0.5–1 mmol/kg ivi.

Table 1 **Features of anaphylactic and anaphylactoid reactions**				
Cardiovascular	**Airway**	**Respiratory**	**Skin**	**General**
Palpitations	Itching of palate or	Bronchospasm	Erythema	Nausea,
Collapse	external auditory		Generalized	vomiting,
Shock	meatus		pruritis	abdominal pain
	Rhinitis		Urticaria	Sense of
	Laryngeal oedema		Conjunctivitis	impending doom
	Angio-oedema			Fainting
				lightheadedness
				Loss of
				consciousness

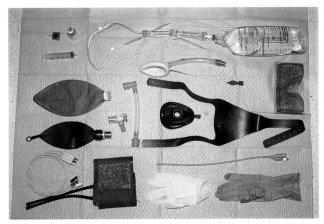

Fig. 3 **See clinical case 33.**

Clinical case 33

In your opinion, which of the products in Fig. 3 contain latex?
See comment on page 125.

Allergic reactions

- Allergic reactions are life-threatening immune responses to foreign substances.
- Always enquire about a history of allergies.
- The diagnosis is clinical usually involving cardiorespiratory compromise.
- Adrenaline (epinephrine) 0.5 mg im is indicated in severe cases.

Shock

Shock refers to inadequate tissue perfusion or blood flow, of which there are several causes in the perioperative period. Physicians should understand the various causes and manifestations of shock as accurate diagnosis of the underlying problem guides appropriate management. Shock is distinct from hypoxia in that adequate tissue perfusion does not guarantee sufficient tissue oxygenation. However, any person who has shock or impaired tissue perfusion, will also have tissue hypoxia. Generally, the presentation includes low blood pressure and tachycardia. Elucidating the cause is based on history, examination and investigations.

Flow (cardiac output CO) =

$$\frac{\text{pressure (mean arterial pressure MAP} - \text{central venous pressure CVP)}}{\text{resistance (systemic vascular resistance)}}$$

Flow (CO) = heart rate (HR) × stroke volume (SV)

Hypovolaemic shock

Dehydration and haemorrhage occur frequently with surgery (Fig. 1). The preoperative fluid deficit is compounded by blood loss and accelerated intraoperative dehydration. Hypovolaemia is the commonest cause of shock following surgery. Cardiac filling is impaired leading to a reduction in SV with a resultant decrease in CO. Volume status may be difficult to assess and overzealous rehydration may be inappropriate. Nonetheless, the dangers of persistent hypovolaemia may exceed those of fluid overload.

Cardiogenic shock

Patients frequently have a history of impaired effort tolerance or ischaemic heart disease. Sudden deterioration in cardiac function may occur following a myocardial infarction or the acute onset of an arrhythmia such as atrial fibrillation. The inability of the heart to contract optimally results in decreased SV leading to low CO.

Obstructive shock

It is imperative to identify causes of obstructive shock, as these are frequently reversible. Obstruction may relate to filling of the heart or to flow from the heart. In both instances, CO is compromised.

Tension pneumothorax occurs when air escapes from the lung into the pleural space. Intrathoracic pressure increases to the extent that cardiac filling is impaired. In severe asthma, obstruction to airflow limits expiratory flow and air becomes trapped in the lungs. Again intrathoracic pressure impedes filling of the heart. Cardiac tamponade and constrictive pericarditis prevent optimum cardiac filling, as does pulmonary embolism. Outflow obstruction is a feature of aortic stenosis and hypertophic obstructive cardiomyopathy.

Distributive shock

The systemic inflammatory response syndrome (SIRS) and anaphylactic reactions may result in distributive shock. The diagnosis of SIRS is made clinically. Underlying insults which may result in SIRS include sepsis, pancreatitis, burns, trauma, liver failure, fat embolism, massive blood transfusion and pre-eclampsia.

The features of SIRS are:

- Tachycardia (HR > 90/min).
- Tachypnoea (RR > 20/min).
- Temperature < 35°C or > 38°C.
- White cell count < 4 or > 11 × 10^9/L.

There are usually several mechanisms of impaired perfusion in those with distributive shock. Vascular tone is decreased following a profound release of endogenous vasodilators, in particular nitric oxide and prostacyclin. Mediators, including cytokines, prostaglandins, proteases, leukotrienes and histamine, lead to increased capillary permeability with resultant loss of intravascular volume. Myocardial depressant factors (e.g. tumour necrosis factor) may also be present, aggravating inadequate tissue perfusion and complicating the clinical picture.

Diagnosis and treatment

Until a specific diagnosis is made, there are a number of useful therapeutic interventions (Fig. 2). If the patient is not responsive, resuscitation for cardiorespiratory arrest should commence. High-flow oxygen and intravenous fluids are the usual initial interventions. If haemorrhage is suspected, emergency (O negative) blood may be indicated.

Other reversible causes, including anaphylaxis, tamponade and tension pneumothorax, should be excluded early and treated appropriately. Central venous pressure (Fig. 3) may help distinguish between hypovolaemic and distributive shock, where CVP is usually low, and cardiogenic shock, where CVP may be elevated. The end-points of treatment for hypovolaemic shock include a normal metabolic acid–base status, adequate urine output, haemoglobin concentration sufficient to support oxygen carriage (Hb > 8 g/dl) and a CVP that increases in response to a fluid challenge.

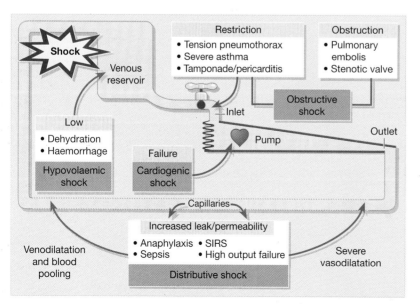

Fig. 1 **Mechanisms of different causes of shock.**

The management of cardiogenic shock is extremely difficult. Not only is perfusion impaired, but pulmonary oedema may also compromise gas exchange and cause hypoxaemia. The cornerstones of therapy include oxygen, a diuretic (typically frusemide), a venodilator (like glygeryl trinatrate), and an inotropic agent (such as epinephrine, dobutamine, dopexamine or a phosphodiesterase inhibitor). Patients should be admitted to a coronary care or intensive care unit for advanced management.

The treatment of anaphylaxis is dealt with on page 75. Distributive shock secondary to a SIRS requires urgent admission to an intensive care unit. Patients usually require tracheal intubation and ventilatory support. Initial management consists both of fluid replacement and inotropes (epinephrine or norepinephrine). Broad-spectrum antimicrobial therapy may be indicated,

unless specific organisms have been detected in blood cultures, in which case therapy may be targeted specifically. These patients frequently develop multiple organ dysfunction including acute respiratory distress syndrome (ARDS), renal failure and myocardial dysfunction. The priority is supportive treatment until intensive care is available.

Scenarios

The various causes of shock may have similar clinical manifestations,

emphasizing the need for directed history, examination and investigations to discriminate among them.

Common clinical presentation

A 60-year-old man has undergone coronary artery bypass surgery. Following surgery he is sweating and confused with a heart rate of 120 bpm and a blood pressure of 85/40 mmHg. Urine output has been steadily tailing off. See Tables 1–4 for possible scenarios for this patient.

Table 1 Scenario 1: hypovolaemic shock (haemorrhage)

History	Examination	Investigations
Good preoperative effort tolerance	Pale	Hb = 6.5 g/dl
Difficulty achieving haemostasis intraoperatively	Peripherally shut down	Urea = 16 mmol/l
Significant blood loss following surgery	CVP = 2 cmH₂O	Creatinine = 140 μmol/l
Postoperative hypothermia		Concentrated urine

Table 2 Scenario 2: distributive (septic) shock

History	Examination	Investigations
The patient is a smoker	Pyrexial, tachypnoeic, cyanosed	Elevated white cell count
He took longer than normal to wean off mechanical ventilation	Warm peripheries with bounding pulses	Blood culture – gram-negative bacilli
	Chest – crackles and bronchial breathing R lower zone.	CXR – RLL consolidation
	Coughing copious secretions	Bronchial secretions – *Klebsiella* species
	CVP = 8 cmH₂O	

Table 3 Scenario 3: obstructive shock (cardiac tamponade)

History	Examination	Investigations
The patient was well preoperatively	Distended neck veins, hypotension and distant heart sounds (Beck's triad)	ECG – small complexes
The operation went well	Marked pulsus paradoxus (20 mmHg)	Echocardiorophy – fluid in the pericardium

Table 4 Scenario 4: cardiogenic shock

History	Examination	Investigations
Poor preoperative effort tolerance	Oedematous	CXR – cardiomegaly and diffuse basal infiltrates
Ejection fraction < 30%	Basal crackles in the chest	
Previous episodes of heart failure	Displaced apex beat	Echo – confirms poor cardiac function
Patient has received 3 L of 5% dextrose water	Third heart sound	
	CVP = 22 cmH₂O.	

Clinical case 34

A 55-year-old heavy smoker has lost about 1000 ml of blood following surgery. He is pale, cold and clammy with a blood pressure of 90/50 mmHg and heart rate is 120 bpm. The CVP is 8 cmH₂O, which is within the normal range. Does this exclude hypovolaemia?
See comment on page 125.

Shock

- Shock is inadequate tissue perfusion.

- Shock may be classified according to the underlying cause: hypovolaemic, cardiogenic, obstructive or distributive.

- Hypovolaemic shock is the most common following surgery.

- The clinical manifestations of the different types of shock may be similar.

- Initial emergency management includes oxygen and intravenous fluids.

Clinical diagnosis of shock

Immediate management:
- Airway/Breathing/Circulation
- Administer oxygen
- Administer fluids
- Blood for FBC, chemistry and cross match

Response — Good → **Continue support**
- Blood and volume
- Exclude bleeding
- Check ABG
- Check coag.

Response — Poor

Consider
- Anaphylaxis, asthma pneumothorax, tamponade

Advanced management
- Invasive monitoring
- Inotropic support
- Ventilatory support
- Intensive care

Fig. 2 **Treatment algorithm.**

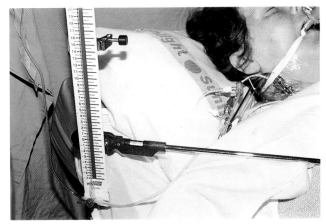

Fig. 3 **A central line attached to a water manometer.**

Pain assessment

If a scholar has neither the conceptual framework nor the methodological training to evaluate a phenomenon, he or she is not likely to consider it. Post and Robins, 1993

Pain is the most common reason for a patient attending the doctor. It is a complex, multidimensional symptom determined not only by tissue injury and nociception but by a variety of cultural, situational and psychological factors.

Factors influencing pain experience

- Age
- Gender
- Personality
- Culture
- Learned behaviour/past experience
- Beliefs/attitudes
- Religion/spirituality
- Anxiety/fears

Assessment

In order to undertake a relevant and worthwhile pain assessment, you must take time to develop good listening and questioning skills. Believing the patient and establishing rapport are of great importance.

Assessment of pain requires:

- A detailed history.
- A comprehensive physical examination.
- An understanding of pain pathophysiology.
- Methodical documentation.
- Pain measurement (using a pain assessment tool).

Pain history

Questioning should identify the location, intensity and temporal nature of the pain. Where possible an assessment of the effects of pain on behaviour and emotional stability should be included. This later part of the assessment can be difficult as patients may be unaware of, or reluctant to discuss, such issues. Many people still (wrongly) view pain as a purely physical problem.

Physical examination: look, feel, move

It is important not to limit the examination to just the painful area, as the pain experienced may be referred,

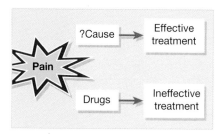

Fig. 1 **Physical examination should lead to effective treatment.**

resulting in the true origin of the pain being overlooked. (see Fig. 1).

Timing of assessment

Ideally pain should be assessed both at rest and on movement/function. Pain at rest may be easy to improve but pain on function, e.g. coughing or movement, may be a more realistic and useful measurement to make.

Pain pathophysiology

Taking a complete history and performing a detailed examination can point towards the aetiology of the pain. It should be possible to determine whether the pain is acute or chronic; somatic, visceral or psychogenic in origin and neuropathic or nociceptive in nature. For details of the pathophysiology of pain see pages 80–81.

Methods of pain assessment

Using an observer

Pain is subjective and a highly individual experience; where possible its assessment should be made by the person experiencing the pain. However there are times where this can be very difficult e.g. early in the postoperative period when the patient is drowsy and in the very young. In these situations, observer alertness to non-verbal cues such as restlessness, crying, grimacing, lacrimation, hypertension and hyperventilation, although not specific to pain, can alert the carer to the fact that the patient may be experiencing pain.

Patient scoring systems

Scoring scales are of value both to quantify and measure pain intensity. They can also help assess analgesic efficacy and the effectiveness of treatment interventions. When opioid analgesics have been given, an assessment of sedation level should be recorded simultaneously.

Example of a sedation score:

- 0 = awake
- 1 = drowsy
- 2 = asleep but rousable
- 3 = unrousable

Table 1 **Pain assessment and measurement considerations**	
History (SIDEARM mnemonic)	
Site	Where is the pain?
Intensity	Is it mild/moderate/severe?
Duration	How long have you had it?
	Acute or gradual onset?
	Intermittent or constant?
Elsewhere	Does the pain radiate anywhere else?
Associated factors	How has the pain affected your sleep pattern, mood, lifestyle?
Relieving factors	What can you do that makes the pain better?
Management to date	Have you had any tests/treatments for the pain? What did they show? How well did the treatment work?
Examination	
Look:	
Patient	Facial expression, abnormal posture or movement, tachycardic, hyptertensive, sweating?
Site	Infection, inflammation, muscle-wasting, bruising?
Feel	Avoid causing the patient pain!
	Normal or abnormal sensation? Diminished or enhanced?
Move	Response to active and passive movement?
	Stiffness? Limitation?
Measurement and documentation	
Listen and believe	
Choose appropriate assessment tool for patient	Adult or child? Drowsy or confused?
Choose appropriate assessment tool for the pain	Unidimensional or multidimensional?
Measure at rest and on movement	
Sedation score required?	
Reassess frequently	Tailor treatment to each finding

Table 2 **Examples of scoring systems**

	Verbal rating score	Numerical rating score	Visual analogue scale	McGill Pain Questonnaire
Example	0 = No pain 1 = Mild pain 2 = Moderate pain 3 = Severe pain	Please indicate the number between 0 and 10 which best describes your pain: 0=no pain/10= worst pain imaginable	10 cm line: no pain to worst pain Patient marks line at appropriate point e.g. no pain _____ worst pain Patient's mark ← 10 cm →	20 sets of words that describe pain of varying intensity Also combines verbal rating score and scale of present pain intensity
Pros	Simple and easy for patient to use Concise + quick Can be used comparatively Good for: ward-based assessments, acute pain, postoperative pain	As for verbal rating scores plus: increased scale allows for more potential discrimination in pain intensity Easily adapted for children 'Hurt themometers'	As for verbal rating scores plus: reproducible, recognized research tool Sensitive assessment May be extrapolated to 'ratios of pain' (allowing analysis by parametric and nonparametric statistics)	Assesses multidimensional aspects of pain: sensory, intensity, affective, evaluative More sensitive than unidimensional Established research tool Good for chronic pain
Cons	Unidimensional Limited to 4 categories Limited research application	Unidimensional	Unidimensional May be difficult for elderly, visually impaired, sedated and young children to use	Time-consuming Rank order words have rank order scale values which assume equal step in intensity, which may not be the case Available words may not fit patient's pain

Pain measurement and assessment tools

The assessment tool must be appropriate to the patient (i.e. a child will require a different tool from an adult), and appropriate for the type of pain (i.e. acute or chronic).

Quantitative pain measurement tools

These assessment systems require the patient to provide a single numerical value to the pain that they are experiencing, either on a continuous or interval scale. Tools can be unidimensional, measuring only one aspect of the pain e.g. intensity, or multidimensional, encompassing several components e.g. pain intensity, sleep disturbance, activity level, mood (Fig. 2).

Qualitative pain measurement tools

More complex scoring systems were developed to provide a more sensitive and discriminative assessment. The McGill Pain Questionnaire (MPG) and the Brief Pain Inventory are frequently used for multidimensional testing, assessing pain in three dimensions: sensory, affective and evaluative. Questionnaires like the MPG are widely used, especially in chronic pain and palliative care settings however, some criticisms have been made (Table 2).

Remember that the patient's satisfaction about pain relief, although not quantitative, may be as important as any actual measurement that has been recorded.

Fig. 2 **Brief pain inventory. Source Pain Reasearch Group, Department of Neurology, University of Wisconsin–Madison. Multidimensional Pain Assessment Tool.**

Assessing pain

- Consider the cause of pain (using history and physical examination findings).
- Assess the pain (using an appropriate tool for the type of patient and type of pain, involve both patient and observer).
- Choose an appropriate method of analgesia (as indicated by the pathophysiological nature of the pain).
- Regularly assess, measure and document pain at rest and on movement (listening to and believing what the patient says).
- Review and refine treatment constantly (as indicated by the patient's assessments).
- Consider possible interaction between pain and non-physiological factors, which may need treated separately.

Pain definitions and physiology

Pain is a widespread problem and a common presenting symptom in both general practice and in hospital medicine. Both physiological and psychological components influence how much pain is felt (intensity) and how we react to the experience of pain. These components can be further subdivided into:

- Sensory – the neural detection of noxious stimuli (physiological component).
- Cognitive – the thoughts associated with pain (psychological component).
- Affective – emotional reactions to pain, such as feeling depressed (psychological component).
- Behavioural – what actions or avoidance techniques are employed to help cope or deal with the pain (psychological component).

The terminology used to describe pain can be confusing. Table 1 contains a list of some of the more commonly used pain terms and a brief explanation of their meaning.

Physiological component

One of the most important functions of the nervous system is to provide information about the threat of bodily harm. The body's neural detection of pain is called nociception.

Nociception involves the relay of information peripherally from special receptors in the tissues (nociceptors) to central structures within the brain.

The pain system has several components (see Fig. 1):

- Specialized receptors called nociceptors, in the peripheral nervous system, detect and filter the intensity and type of noxious stimuli.
- Primary afferent fibres (A-delta and C fibres) transmit noxious stimuli to the CNS.
- Dorsal horn area of the spinal cord is where the primary afferent fibres synapse with second-order neurons and where complex interconnections take place between local excitatory and inhibitory interneurons and the descending inhibitory tracts from the brain.
- Ascending nociceptive tracts (e.g. the spinothalamic tract) relay the signal to higher centres in the CNS.
- Higher centres are involved in pain discrimination, the affective components of pain, pain memory and pain-related motor responses (i.e. withdrawal response).
- Descending inhibitory systems modify incoming nociceptive impulses at spinal cord level.

Psychological component

Nociception is not directly translated into pain sensation. The spinal cord is

Table 1	**Definitions of terms**
Term	**Definition**
Pain	An unpleasant sensory and emotional experience associated with actual or potential tiissue damage, or described in such terms (IASP definition)
Pain threshold	Minimum stimulus required to produce cortical response on 50% of occasions, mediated by A-delta fibres
Pain tolerance	Maximum noxious stimulation patient will tolerate, mediated by C fibres
Allodynia	Painful response to non-painful stimulus
Hyperalgesia	Increased response to painful stimulus, mediated by sensitized polymodal receptors
Primary hyperalgesia	Hyperalgesia at the site of injury
Secondary hyperalgesia	Hyperalgesia in the surrounding skin
Pre-emptive analgesia	Administration of analgesic agent before noxious stimulus to prevent sensitization of the dorsal horn
Receptive field	Peripheral area from which neural stimulation will elicit a neurophysiological response in a central neuron
Sensitization	Increased activity in a nerve as a result of alteration of the chemical environment or action of other nerves
Wind-up	Change in the activity of the dorsal horn area of the spinal cord, as a result of persistent C fibre stimulation (neuroplasticity)

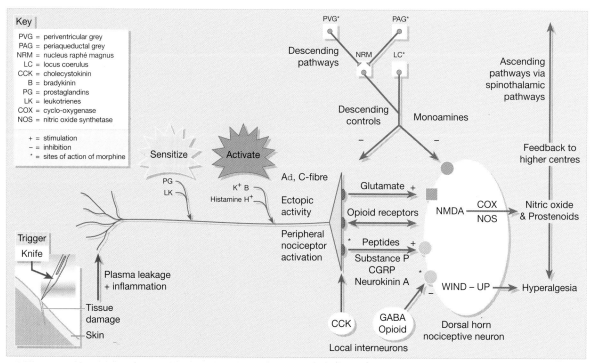

Fig. 1 **The physiology of pain.**

capable of amplifying or suppressing the transmission of nociception to the brain. This means that a person's psychological state can affect their sensation of pain, as well as their emotional and behavioural responses. This is the rationale behind using psychological approaches such as distraction therapy and relaxation techniques in the management of pain.

Types of pain are nociceptive, neuropathic and psychogenic.

Nociceptive pain

This type of pain arises from tissue damage (somatic or visceral). The release of inflammatory mediators from tissues, immune cells and sympathetic and sensory nerve endings results in direct or indirect stimulation of nociceptors (see Fig. 1). Two types of signal are transmitted as a consequence of this nociceptor activation:

1) Physiological (fast) pain is due to stimulation of high-threshold thermo/mechanical nociceptors (Meissner's corpuscles, Meckel's discs). This pain is protective in function, causing an immediate withdrawal from the stimulus to prevent further damage. It is transmitted via fast-conducting A-delta (Aδ) primary afferent neurons which synapse with secondary neurons in the dorsal horn of the spinal cord. If the stimulus is of short duration and there is no tissue damage, the pain disappears when the stimulus disappears.

2) Pathophysiological (slow) pain is responsible for the delayed pain sensation that occurs after tissue injury and which encourages tissue healing by eliciting behaviour to protect the damaged area. This is the type of pain that occurs after surgery, trauma and inflammation and is the kind that doctors try to manage clinically. High-threshold polymodal nociceptors respond to mechanical, thermal and chemical stimuli and transmit their signal to the dorsal horn via slow-conducting C fibres. Stimulated C fibres release peptides which sensitize low-threshold nociceptors, resulting in peripheral sensitization at the site of injury (primary hyperalgesia).

The dorsal horn

Melzack and Wall proposed the Gate Theory of Pain in 1965. This theory proposed that pain pathways (Aδ and C) can be blocked by the stimulation of touch fibres (Aβ) which inhibit transmission to ascending pathways via an interneuron in the substantia gelatinosa.

It is now known that the central nervous system is not hard-wired as the above theory originally proposed, but is capable of adapting. C fibres, if triggered by a stimulus to fire ≥ 3 seconds, give rise to slow temporal summation, where the intensity of the pain increases with every repeat stimulation, despite the stimulus remaining at the same intensity. This phenomenon is known as *wind-up* (see Table 1). Wind-up produces a widening of the peripheral receptive field which exhibits exaggerated responses to noxious stimuli and an increased rate of spontaneous discharge (secondary hyperalgesia).

Several different receptors and neurotransmitters are involved in the pain pathway at dorsal horn level and this makes the dorsal horn an especially important target for the action of analgesic agents (Table 2).

Neuropathic pain

Neuropathic pain is caused by injury to the nerve pathway. This can lead to intact neurons in close proximity to the damaged nerve sprouting and growing into the denervated area, resulting in the development of *allodynia* (see Table 1).

The stimuli producing this allodynia may be mechanical, or due to spontaneous firing or to increased sensitivity to noradrenaline, the latter resulting in sympathetically maintained pain (SMP). SMP is often a component of the chronic pain condition known as complex regional pain syndrome (CRPS) (see 'Chronic pain syndromes', pages 92–93). Neuropathic pain often responds poorly to conventional analgesics and patients with this type of pain frequently need to be referred for specialist treatment at a pain clinic.

Psychogenic pain

Psychogenic pain constitutes a small but important group of patients with pain, where pain and anxiety or depression co-exist. However, it is often difficult to differentiate whether pain is secondary to or the actual cause of the psychological problem.

This multifaceted character of pain and its subjective nature can often make pain difficult to assess in an objective way.

Table 2 **Important targets for the action of analgesic agents**

Target	Action	Pharmacological intervention
Periphery		
Prostaglandins (PG)	Sensitize nociceptor	Non-steroidal anti-inflammatory drugs (NSAIDs) e.g. aspirin
Primary afferent sensory nerve	Pain transmission	Local anaesthetic nerve block
Dorsal horn		
Opioid receptors (pre- and post-synaptic)	Inhibit pain transmission	Opioid agonist: Endogenous e.g. endorphin; Exogenous e.g. morphine
NMDA receptor	Secondary hyperalgesia Chronic pain states	NMDA receptor antagonist, e.g. ketamine
GABA receptor	Inhibits pain transmission	GABA receptor agonist, e.g. baclofen
Higher centres		
Opioid receptors (pre- and post-synaptic)	Inhibit pain transmission	Opioid agonist, e.g. morphine
Descending systems		
Adrenergic (α_2) receptors	Inhibit pain transmission	Endogenous = noradrenaline Exogenous: direct = clonidine, indirect = amitriptyline
Serotonic receptors	Inhibit pain transmission	α_2- adrenergic + serotonic agonist, e.g. tramadol

Pain definitions and physiology

- Pain is a complex sensation incorporating physiological, psychological and social factors and treatment should address all of these components.
- The human nervous system is dynamic and readily adapts to a changing environment, sometimes in a protective way, i.e. with nociceptive pain, or in a non-beneficial way, i.e. neuropathic pain.
- Understanding pain physiology promotes effective pharmacological targeting and adoption of a multimodal therapeutic approach.
- Relieving pain is important for humanitarian reasons but if analgesia is given pre-emptively, it may prevent wind-up occuring in the dorsal horn and reduce the incidence of chronic pain states developing.

Pharmacological intervention in pain management

The methods used to manage pain must take into account the multidimensional nature of the problem, addressing the sensory, affective, cognitive and behavioural components. Remember that while drugs have an important role in the management of pain, physical and psychological techniques should also be considered.

The key to optimising analgesia is to treat the individual and provide appropriate analgesia for the severity of pain. The World Health Organization introduced a step-like ladder as a guide to analgesia prescribing in cancer patients (see 'Cancer pain management' on page 100 for diagram). It provides a useful framework for prescribing analgesia for most painful conditions.

In general, analgesic drugs commonly used to treat pain can be classified as follows:

- Non-opioid analgesics (e.g. paracetamol, NSAIDs).
- Opioid analgesics (e.g. morphine and its derivatives).
- Adjuvant analgesics (e.g. antidepressants, anticonvulsants, alpha-2 agonists).

Non-opioid analgesics

Paracetamol (acetaminophen)
Paracetamol has been widely used since the mid 1950s as an analgesic and antipyretic. Its mechanism of action is unclear, but it is thought to inhibit the production of prostaglandins centrally. Unlike NSAIDs, paracetamol has very little action on peripheral cyclo-oxygenase activity and does not possess anti-inflammatory action. In recommended therapeutic doses paracetamol is well tolerated in both children and adults, with few side-effects, however large doses (> 8 g) usually consumed as an intentional overdose, may cause potentially fatal hepatic necrosis.

Non-steroidal anti-inflammatory drugs (NSAIDs)
The NSAIDs possess analgesic, anti-inflammatory, antiplatelet and antipyretic effects. NSAIDs are being used increasingly in the perioperative and early postoperative period for minor and superficial surgery and are playing a significant role as co-analgesics following major surgery (see Table 1). NSAIDs used in conjunction with opioid medication following major surgery can reduce opioid requirements by as much as one third over the first 2 postoperative days.

NSAIDs – mechanism of action
Tissue damage and inflammation lead to local synthesis, via cyclo-oxygenase (COX), of prostaglandins which stimulate nociceptors and sensitize them to other inflammatory mediators, such as bradykinin and histamine. Aspirin and all other NSAIDs inhibit the COX enzyme in peripheral tissue, reducing prostaglandin-induced inflammation and sensitization of primary afferent sensory neurones. Aspirin *irreversibly* blocks cyclo-oxygenase activity, within 1 hour of administration, by acetylating serine 530 at the active site of the enzyme. All the other NSAIDs *reversibly* inhibit COX. NSAIDs are also thought to have a central effect as an antipyretic, mediated through the hypothalamus.

NSAIDs can be classified according to their chemical structure, e.g. salicylates, acetic acids, propionic acids. NSAIDs are well absorbed in the gastrointestinal tract and are usually administered orally or rectally; some preparations can be given parenterally. Unlike opioids, NSAIDS produce no respiratory depression and lack the potential for physical dependence. However an analgesic ceiling effect has been demonstrated for all NSAIDs, independent of route of administration, after which the incidence of adverse side-effects escalates (Table 1).

Methods for reducing side-effects of NSAIDs
Empirical use of various prophylactic therapies such as antacids, sucralfate, H$_2$ blockers, omeprazole.

Misoprostol, a prostaglandin synthetic analogue. A preparation containing both diclofenac sodium (50 mg or 75 mg) and misoprostol (200 ug) is currently available on the market.

COX isoenzymes – two forms of the COX enzyme occur in the body (isoenzymes). COX-1 is responsible for the production of the prostaglandins which regulate cytoprotection (e.g. gastric mucosal protection) and cellular homeostasis (e.g. kidney function, PGE2 and haemostatic function, endothelial PGI2, platelets, thromboxane A2). COX-2 is expressed only after tissue trauma or when triggered by pro-inflammatory agents like cytokines, bradykinin and histamine.

NSAIDs block COX-1 and COX-2 to different extents. The ratio of potency against COX-1 and potency against COX-2 explains the efficacy/side-effect profile of each NSAID (see Table 2).

In 1996, the first drug to be marketed as a specific COX-2 inhibitor (Meloxicam) was launched in the UK, with potential benefits for providing anti-inflammatory, antipyrexial and analgesic effects with a reduced potential for producing serious gastrointestinal and renal side-effects. Several newer COX-2 inhibiting agents are now also available.

Opioid analgesics

Opioid analgesics are a large family of compounds, which differ in their potency, duration of action and side-effects. They

Table 1 Indications, contraindications and side-effects of NSAIDs

Indications	Contraindications	Major side-effects
Acute pain, mild to moderate	Hypersensitivity to NSAIDs (esp. asthmatics)	Gastric irritation + ulceration
Rheumatoid and osteoarthritis	History of bleeding ulcers	Haemostatic impairment
Myalgia	Haemophilia	Increased bleeding time
Neuralgia	Renal disease	CNS toxicity, headache, tinnitus
Prophylactic treatment of CVS and thrombotic-related illness		Aspirin-induced asthma
		Renal complications

Table 2 The potency ratio against COX-1 and COX-2 for common NSAIDs

NSAID	Potency ratio (Cox-1:Cox-2 inhibition)
Diclofenac	1:1
Ibuprofen	0.2:1
Aspirin	50:1

produce their effect by acting on specific opioid receptors. Three main opioid receptor subclasses have been identified – mu (μ), kappa (κ) and delta (δ). There are important differences between the effects elicited by receptor activation (Table 3).

Most opioids are agonists at the mu receptor, found in the central nervous system and in the periphery. Morphine and diamorphine are examples of pure opioid receptor agonists and have a strong analgesic action. Codeine, dextropropoxyphene and dihydrocodeine are also mu-receptor agonists but have weak analgesic action, either dose-limited by side-effects (e.g. constipation with codeine) or by their lower binding affinity for the mu receptor (e.g. dextropropoxyphene). The potency of an opioid may vary with pain type (nociceptive or neuropathic), renal function and with previous opioid exposure. As a result of this, theoretical equi-analgesic doses should only be used as an approximate guide when switching patients to another opioid (Table 4).

Compound preparations incorporating paracetamol are available but can contain a low, sometimes subtherapeutic dose of the weak opioid, e.g. cocodamol can contain only 8 mg of codeine (recommended therapeutic dose for codeine is 30–40 mg). It may be more appropriate to prescribe the drugs separately in their full analgesic dose. Some opioids, classified as partial agonists, bind to the opioid receptor without fully stimulating it (e.g. buprenorphine).

One of the major disadvantages of opioid analgesics is their many side-effects:

- Nausea and vomiting is experienced by about 1/3 of patients on opioids.
- Constipation is a problem, particularly in long-term opioid use.
- Drowsiness is common when starting on opioids but appears to diminish over a few days.

- Respiratory depression is an important indicator of opioid toxicity. Remember that it is the respiratory rate that falls rather than the tidal volume.
- Tolerance may develop, especially when opioids are employed long-term, and the dose may have to be reassessed and adjusted at regular intervals.
- Addiction is rarely a problem where physical pain is present.

Reversal of opioid overdosage is best achieved by intravenous naloxone. Naloxone is a relatively selective mu-receptor antagonist. The response is rapid and specific, occurring within 2 minutes of an intravenous bolus of 400–800 μg. As the duration of naloxone is 1–2 hours, shorter than most opioids, further bolus doses of naloxone or a constant infusion may be necessary to maintain clinical improvement.

Adjuvant analgesics

These drugs can produce analgesia but were not originally marketed for this purpose, e.g. antidepressants, anticonvulsants, alpha-2 agonists, such as clonidine and corticosteroids. They tend to be reserved for complex or unresponsive pain states, where they are administered under direct supervision of a specialized pain management team and in chronic or palliative pain states.

Table 3 Opioid receptor sub-classes

Receptor type	Function
mu (μ)	Analgesia, respiratory depression, euphoria, dependence, nausea and vomiting
kappa (κ)	Spinal analgesia, sedation, miosis
delta (δ)	Analgesia, respiratory depression, euphoria, constipation

Table 4 Equi-analgesic doses of opioid

Opioid	Equivalent dose	
	Parental	Oral
Agonist		
Morphine	10 mg	30 mg
Diamorphine	5 mg	60 mg
Pethidine	100 mg	300 mg
Oxycodone	15 mg	20 mg
Fentanyl	100 μg	NA
Hydromorphone	1.5 mg	7.5 mg
Methadone	10 mg	20 mg
Codeine	130 mg	200 mg
Dexthropropoxyphene		130 mg
Tramadol	100 mg	
Partial agonist		
Buprenorphine	0.4 mg	0.4–0.8 mg (sublingual)

Clinical case 35

A 42-year-old woman has arrived back on the ward 2 hours post abdominal hysterectomy. She has an intravenous morphine patient-controlled analgesic (PCA) system attached. You are asked to review her as she is still complaining of severe abdominal pain, which is exacerbated by her frequent retching.
Part 1 Discuss your assessment and management of this case.
Part 2 The PCA bolus dose has been increased to 2 mg. 45 minutes later you are asked to urgently review the same patient as nursing staff are finding it difficult to rouse her. What do you think might be the reason for her present state? How would you treat this problem?
See comment on pages 125–126.

Pharmacological intervention in pain management

- Pharmacological treatment is only one option available to treat pain.
- Treat the cause of the pain (certain types of analgesics are more effective in certain pain states, eg. NSAIDs for inflammatory pain).
- Remember the 'Rule of Fives' when prescribing analgesia:
  - By the mouth
  - By the clock
  - By the ladder
  - For the individual
  - Adjuvant medication.
- Reassess the effect of the treatment and modify as required, watching for signs of toxicity or tolerance developing.

Acute pain management

Acute pain can be defined as pain of recent onset and of limited duration. It usually has a temporal and causal relationship to injury or disease (e.g. postoperative pain, appendicitis, broken arm). Acute pain can have widespread effects on the physiological homeostasis of the body. These effects are shown in Fig. 1 and collectively contribute to the entity known as the stress response. The stress response is covered in more detail on pages 46 and 47.

If acute pain remains untreated for any duration of time, it can lead to an increased risk of postoperative complications, a slower recovery and an increased likelihood of developing chronic pain.

The degree of postoperative pain experienced by individuals following surgery varies greatly. Pain intensity is greatest at the onset of injury and immediately after surgery. However the duration of severe pain is relatively short-lived and normally should be greatly reduced by 48–72 hours postoperatively. Effective analgesia for acute pain is necessary for humanitarian reasons but additional benefits have also been demonstrated.

Benefits of early effective analgesia

- Respiratory function maintenance (decreased incidence of atelectasis, hypoxia and chest infection).
- Early mobilization (decreased incidence of DVT + PTE).
- Reduction in stress response (decreased levels of catecholamines, myocardial work, myocardial ischaemia)
- Psychological benefits (decreased incidence of anxiety).

The severity of the pain experienced depends on many factors. Make a list of as many of these factors that influence pain as you can. (Referring to the 'Pain assessment' on page 78 may help.)

The site of operation is one important factor. Operations that involve thoracic and abdominal incisions, especially where the pleura or peritoneum are breached, will require stronger analgesics than operations with superficial incisions and on the periphery.

Properties of an ideal analgesic agent

- Safe.
- Effective.
- Rapid onset.
- No/minimal side-effects.
- Cheap.
- Easy to store and administer.
- Low abuse potential.

Multimodal analgesia

Multimodal analgesia involves administering a variety of drugs, perhaps given by different routes, to obtain optimal analgesia. NSAIDs, paracetamol, local anaesthetics and opioids have all be used in combination to improve the effectiveness of analgesia in acute pain. Synergism exists between many of the analgesic treatments available, allowing lower doses of component drugs. By administering lower doses of the drugs, the incidence and severity of side-effects and adverse reactions can also be reduced; however, interactions can be a problem. The British National Formulary can be used to identify if a possible interaction is likely.

Methods of analgesia

Pharmacological methods

Analgesia can be administered by a variety of routes (see Table 1). For every analgesic drug, there exists a minimum plasma concentration that must be achieved before an analgesic response to a standard stimulus is obtained. This level is known as the minimum effective analgesic concentration (MEAC).

Physical methods

Physical methods are seldom 100% effective in eliminating pain when used alone and supplementary analgesic medication will also be required.

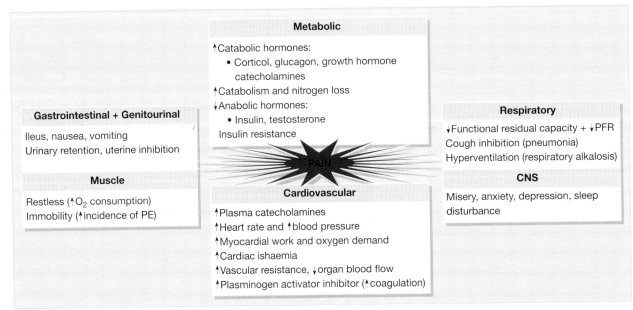

Fig. 1 **Clinical effects of pain**

Table 1 Advantages and disadvantages of various routes of administration

Method of administration	Advantages	Disadvantages
Oral	Convenient and acceptable Painless Relatively Cheap Simple	Absorption/onset slow and variable Limited effectiveness if nausea/vomiting/gastric ileus Some drugs significantly affected by first-pass metabolism, e.g. morphine
Rectal	Avoids gastric irritation Useful if 'nil by mouth' or vomiting	Variable absorption and onset Cultural resistance in UK
Transdermal	Comfortable and well tolerated by patients Avoids oral route Useful for drugs with significant first-pass effect	Suitable for only very lipophilic drugs Great intra- and inter-patient variability for absorption/onset Depot remains in skin when patch removed, possibility of delayed-onset side-effects
Subcutaneous	Cannula may reduce need for painful injections Preserves venous system	Absorption dependent on regional blood flow May produce erythema around injection site
Intramuscular	Cheap	Painful for patients Variable absorption and onset, particularly in the elderly
Intravenous infusion	100% absorption Reliable and fast onset Comfortable for patients	Risk of overdose if not regularly assessed Risk of respiratory depression with opioids Reliable equipment needed
Intravenous bolus	100% absorption, rapid onset Treatment tailored to individual needs	Time-consuming Experienced trained staff required
Intravenous patient-controlled analgesia (see pages 86–87)	100% absorption, rapid onset Individualization of treatment Minimal delay between analgesic demand and administration	Expensive equipment required Intensive monitoring and assessment required
Epidural	Good analgesia at small doses, reducing drug side-effects Reduces risk of DVT and chest infections Reduces stress response to surgery	Requires an anaesthetist to insert Intensive monitoring (depending on hospital policy may require nursed in a HDU or ITU setting) Risk of delayed complications, e.g. urinary retention Potential motor block inadvertently produced
Peripheral nerve blocks	Good analgesia Minimal upset to other body systems	Limited duration Skill required to insert Potential damage to adjacent organs, e.g. pneumothorax with intercostal nerve block

Splinting, traction and immobilization

When acute pain is caused by trauma, physical treatments such as splinting, traction and immobilization can greatly reduce the amount of pain experienced. These methods should only be employed short term as continued inactivity can lead to weakness, stiffness and result in more pain.

Physiotherapy

Physiotherapy has an important role to play in promoting activity and reducing pain. Techniques such as massage, manipulation, superficial heat and deep heat using short wave diathermy or ultrasound have all been beneficially employed.

Transcutaneous electrical nerve stimulation (TENS)

Electricity has been used to treat pain since the Roman times but was first recorded as being used to treat postoperative acute pain in 1973. TENS is most useful in acute pain management when used along with other therapies (synergism).

Psychological methods

Patients who are afraid of surgery or anaesthesia may experience more pain postoperatively as a consequence. It is important to take time to listen to patient's fears and provide a careful explanation of the procedure(s) at a level appropriate for the patient.

The acute pain team

The working party report by the Royal College of Surgeons and the College of Anaesthetists in 1990 advocated that all hospitals where major surgery takes place should set up acute pain teams as a means of improving postoperative analgesia. Over 50% of UK hospitals now provide this type of service. The acute pain team should ideally be multidisciplinary, usually involving anaesthetic, nursing, surgical and pharmacy input.

The functions of the acute pain team include:

- Assessing patients, especially with epidural or PCA modes of analgesia.
- Educating hospital staff in pain assessment and treatment options.
- Auditing current practice and improving the available service.
- Developing analgesia protocols and promoting safe practice.

It is important to remember that acute pain is not confined to postoperative wards, but is a problem faced in many other clinical settings e.g. MI, renal colic, rheumatoid arthritis. Effective pain relief requires flexibility and tailoring of treatment to an individual rather than rigid application of formulae. However, the fundamental principles for managing acute pain remain the same regardless of aetiology. While it may not be possible to completely alleviate all pain, it should be possible to reduce it to, at minimum, a tolerable or comfortable level.

Acute pain management

- Acute pain includes nociceptive, inflammatory, neurogenic and psychological components.
- Acute pain has widespread effects on the physiological homeostasis of the body.
- Acute pain varies greatly between individuals.
- Acute pain management incorporates pharmacological, physical and psychological modalities.
- Effective analgesia should:
  - provide maximum relief of pain
  - have minimal or no side-effects
  - reduce postoperative complications
  - speed recovery
  - reduce the likelihood of developing of chronic pain.

Patient-controlled analgesia

Patient controlled analgesia (PCA) is a popular and widely used method of postoperative pain control, where parenteral opioid analgesia is likely to be required for more than 24 hours (see Table 1).

Table 1 **Patient-controlled analgesia**	
Advantages	**Disadvantages**
Improved pain relief	Equipment cost
Improved patient satisfaction	Trained staff required
Improved mobility	Technique-related mishaps
Eliminates possible delays in	Masking of postoperative complications
obtaining analgesia	Accumulation of metabolites

Proposed reasons why PCA is popular with patients include:

- Avoidance of intramuscular injections.
- Rapid onset of analgesia.
- Preservation of self-control.

There is huge inter-individual variation in analgesic needs; for this reason PCA is an ideal method for the patient needing much more or less than standard. If plasma levels fall below the analgesic threshold, patients can self-titrate opioids to a level of analgesia that is acceptable to them (within the therapeutic window).

Patient selection

Patients must want to and be willing to use the device. An understanding of the concept, including the lockout period, is required for effective use. PCA has been used successfully in children as young as 5 years old and old age is not a contraindication to use, if prescribing guidelines for opioids in the elderly are remembered. Physical limitation of the upper limb may pose a technical problem as pressing the button to deliver the bolus of drug may prove impossible.

PCA devices

Various types of PCA are available, but fall mainly into two cateogories:

- Electronic (Fig. 2a)
- Disposable (Fig. 2b)

Most electronic PCA devices offer the following standard programming options:

Bolus dose – This is the set amount of drug administered each time the patient presses the demand button.

Lockout time – This is the minimum period of time allowed between two good demand doses. If the patient presses the demand button during the set lockout time no additional dose will be given.

Loading dose – This is a 'one off' bolus of drug, usually given to make the patient comfortable immediately postoperatively. The amount given is variable and is determined by the clinician.

Background infusion – This facility, if selected, permits a continuous infusion of opioid, over and above that which the patient demands.

Bolus dose rate – This determines how quickly the bolus dose is administered.

Pump history – Records good/bad demand doses and gives a cumulative total of opioid used.

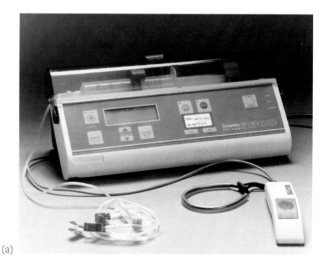
(a)

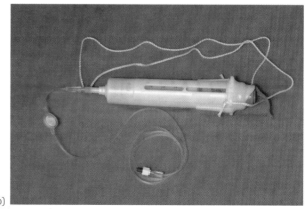
(b)

Fig. 2 **(a) Electronic (Graseby 3300) and (b) disposable (Vygon Freedom 5) PCA devices.**

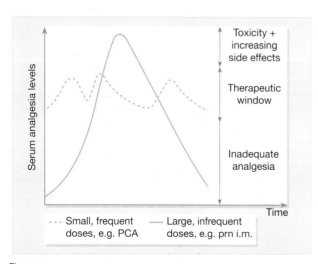

Fig. 1 **Intravenous PCA versus im 'as required' analgesia.** Adapted from Key Facts in Pain by Dr S Peat, Churchill Communications, Europe 1995

Prescribing

The most common opioid analgesics administered by PCA are morphine, diamorphine and pethidine, although fentanyl, tramadol and papaveretum are also used. Anti-emetics can be added to the PCA opioid syringe, e.g. droperidol or metoclopramide, although debate is still ongoing whether these agents should be given as prophylaxis or therapeutically.

The most popular route for PCA is intravenously but the subcutaneous route is gaining in popularity. Patients who have an epidural catheter in situ can also benefit from a form of PCA. A patient-controlled epidural analgesia (PCEA) system can be set up, allowing patients to give themselves a pre-set bolus of local anaesthetic when needed. The PCEA devices used are similar (and in some cases identical) to those used for iv/sc PCA and the same programme options can be applied. Changes to a PCEA, however, must only be made by an anaesthetist or by a member of the Acute Pain Team. Different types of problems occur relating to this method of analgesia and these are discussed in 'Complications' on pages 102–103.

A reasonable starting prescription for an intravenous PCA with morphine (1 mg/ml) would be:

- Bolus dose = 1 mg
- Bolus dose rate = stat.
- Lockout time = 5 minutes
- *Background infusion = 0 mg/hour.

For a diamorphine (2 mg/ml) subcutaneous PCA, a suitable regimen would be:

- Bolus dose = 2 mg
- Bolus dose rate = 5 minutes
- Lockout time = 10 minutes
- *Background infusion = 0 mg/hour.

* Using a continuous background infusion in addition to bolus dosing has been shown to improve analgesia in children, but in adults is often associated with increased side effects (respiratory depression, nausea and vomiting). For this reason, in the majority of cases, a background infusion is not routinely used in the adult population.

Monitoring and safety

PCA devices should be administered through good venous access with connections kept visible (see Fig. 3). If a dedicated intravenous line is not used then the addition of a one-way valve must be used to prevent backflow of opioid into the infusion bag. Pumps should sit below chest height and be orientated horizontally to reduce accidental risk of syphoning. Where portable pumps that hang round the neck are in use, patients should remove the device before sleep to eliminate potential cord strangulation.

Mandatory recordings are required to ensure the safe and effective use of PCA.

- Pain scores (see 'Pain assessment' on pages 78–79).
- Sedation score (see 'Pain assessment' on pages 78–79).
- Respiratory rate.

Pulse oximeter application is encouraged when a PCA is attached. Limits should be set for the above recordings and instructions given for when they fall outwith the given range, i.e. discontinue PCA, give Naloxone 400 μg, call the anaesthetist. See 'Useful advice to house officers and non-anaesthetists' on pages 102–103, for advice on how to trouble-shoot problems encountered with in adults PCAs.

Ward staff should be adequately trained in the principles of PCA and familiar with the pump systems used in their hospital. Hourly assessments as outlined above should be made and changes implemented and documented swiftly where inadequate pain relief is identified.

Some but not all of the PCA devices incorporate a lock device around the syringe. Not only does this prevent accidental/intentional excessive bolus administration but provides a degree of security – a syringe with 100 mg of diamorphine is a valuable commodity!

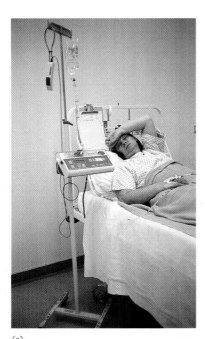
(a)

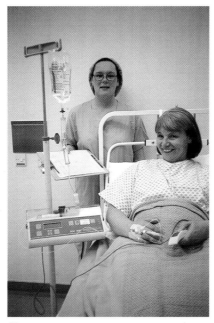
(b)

Fig. 3 **(a) Incorrect and (b) correct PCA set-ups (see Clinical case 36).**

Clinical case 36

See Fig. 3(a) of a patient with a PCA attached. Can you identify 5 faults in this picture?
See comment on page 126.

Patient-controlled analgesia

The key to successful use of PCA is:

- Careful patient selection, ensuring good understanding of use.
- Meticulous programming with appropriate settings.
- Staff familiar with system.
- Frequent pain assessments and drug reappraisal.

Local anaesthesia

Local anaesthetics (LAs) prevent pain by causing a reversible block of conduction along nerve fibres. In order for these drugs to work, they must gain access to the inside of the axon; to do this they must be in a non-ionized (lipophilic) form. Once inside the axon, some of the molecules re-ionize, according to the Henderson–Hasselbach equation, to maintain electrochemical equilibrium. These ionized molecules block the sodium channels of the axon, preventing action potential generation.

Pharmacology

LAs can be divided into amides and esters, depending on their structure (see Fig. 1).

Most of the LAs in current use are amides. Amides precipitate fewer allergic reactions than esters. In general, complications with amides are due to the systemic effects of the drugs, although reactions can occasionally occur due to methylparaben, a preservative found in some amide LAs.

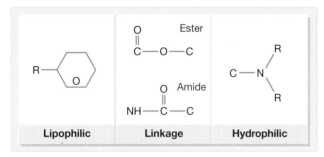

Fig. 1 **Ester/amide linkage of local anaesthetics.**

Clinical applications

Topical administration

EMLA® (**e**utectic **m**ixture of **l**ocal **a**naesthetic) cream and amethocaine gel are effective in relieving the pain associated with needling procedures, such as venepuncture, venous cannulation and lumbar punctures.

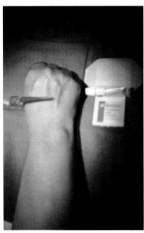
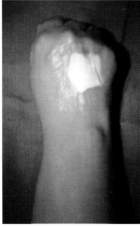

(a)   (b)

Fig. 2 **(a) Identify vein, (b) apply EMLA and cover with occlusive dressing.**

Solid lignocaine and prilocaine mixed in equal proportions undergo a phase-change to a liquid at room temperature, the resultant mixture is known as a 'eutectic' mixture. EMLA cream® consists of a eutectic mixture of 2.5% lignocaine and 2.5% prilocaine in an emulsifier. The concentration of LA in the droplets of the emulsion is 80%, permitting an effective high concentration of LA to be in contact with the skin, while the overall concentration of LA remains relatively low at only 5%.

To be effective the cream should to be applied for a minimum time of one hour. The duration of action once the cream has been removed is 30 to 60 minutes. Blanching of the skin is commonly seen after EMLA® application and should not be regarded as an allergic reaction (see Fig. 2).

The main concern using EMLA® relates to the potential risk of developing methaemoglobinaemia. Methaemoglobin (MetHb) is formed by the oxidation of the ferrous iron in haemoglobin to the ferric state. Two metabolites of prilocaine (4-hydroxy-2-methanylaniline and 2-methlyaniline (ortho-toludine)) have been shown to cause methaemoglobinaemia. Clinically, levels of MetHb above 5% are thought significant as MetHb has very low oxygen-carrying capacity.

- **Be aware of the possibility of accumulation of MetHb with repeated applications of EMLA® cream, especially in infants and neonates**

Amethocaine, available as a topical gel preparation, can be used as an alternative to EMLA®. Its onset time, at 30–40 minutes, is faster than EMLA®, as it is more lipophilic and crosses the stratum corneum barrier more easily. Amethocaine does not cause MetHb and is not associated with hypersensitivity reactions following repeat applications, but itch and mild localized oedema have been documented.

Other methods of LA application:

- Infiltration.
- Nerve block.
- Epidural.
- Subarachnoid.
- Plexus block.
- Single-shot technique.
- Continuous technique (in situ catheter).

More details about these techniques can be found in 'Regional anaesthesia' on pages 90–91.

Choice of drug

Physicochemical properties can influence LA activity in the following ways:

- Greater lipid solubility = higher potency
- Greater protein binding = longer duration
- pKa influences the onset of action. The pKa of a drug is the pH at which ionized and un-ionized forms of a drug are present in equal amounts. Onset of action is directly related to the amount of un-ionized drug present. The percentage of LA present in the unionised form when injected into tissues inversely proportional to the pKa of that agent.

Factors affecting systemic absorption

Site of injection

Local vascularity and the presence of tissue and fat influence the rate of uptake and removal from specific sites. In general, absorption rate decreases in the following order:

Interpleural > Intercostal > Caudal > Epidural > Brachial plexus > Femoral sciatic > Subcutaneous > Intra-articular > Spinal

Dosage factors

The onset time of LA can be decreased by using a higher concentration or a larger volume of the drug and by injecting the LA more rapidly. However it is always better to inject LA drugs slowly as it is more pleasant for the patient, and if an allergic reaction or inadvertent intravascular injection occurs, a smaller drug load will have been given.

Maximum safe dosages (mg/kg) have been calculated for the LAs currently in use (Table 1).

Addition of vasoconstrictors

Co-administering a vasoconstrictor with LA reduces blood flow to the area. Less systemic absorption of the LA occurs, allowing more LA to be given and the overall duration of LA action is prolonged.

Adrenaline and felypressin are two agents used as vasoconstrictors. LA drugs with adrenaline should never be administered near end arteries (e.g. toes, fingers, penis) due to the risk of inducing necrosis at the periphery.

Condition of the patient

Liver disease

Ester LA are broken down by plasma cholinesterases and amide LAs are metabolized by hepatic enzymes. Failure to metabolize the drug will result in higher plasma levels accumulating.

Cardiac failure

Cardiovascular disease may alter the pharmacokinetics of LAs by decreasing the clearance and volume of distribution of the drug.

Concurrent medication

The presence of other drugs which are protein-bound may result in higher plasma concentrations of free LA being available.

Potential problems

All local anaesthetics depress excitable tissue (e.g. myocardium). At high plasma levels clinical signs are manifest in the central nervous (CNS), cardiovascular (CVS) and respiratory (RS) systems (see Fig. 3).

Treatment of systemic toxicity is outline in Fig. 4.

Table 1 Maximum safe dosages of common local anaesthetics		
Drug	Dose (mg/kg)	+Adrenaline (mg/kg)
Lignocaine	3	7
Prilocaine	4	7
Ropivacaine	2	2
Bupivacaine	2	2

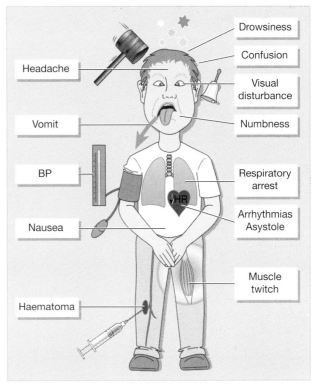

Fig. 3 **Signs and symptoms of local anaesthetic systemic toxicity.**

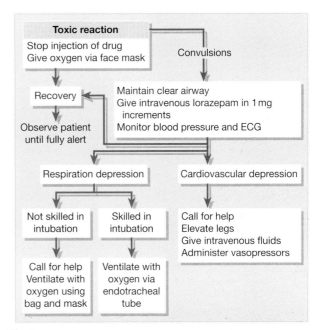

Fig. 4 **Algorithm for the treatment of clinical toxicity.**

Local anaesthetics

- Local anaesthetics (LA) are a versatile and clinically useful group of drugs, which act by causing a reversible block of nerve fibre conduction.

- LA can be given by a variety of routes and are available in cream, gel, tablet and liquid forms.

- Co-administration of LAs with a vasoconstrictor can reduce systemic absorption, allowing more LA to be given, but must never be administered near end-arteries (e.g. toes, fingers, penis).

- The maximum safe dosage of LA should not be exceeded, as systemic toxicity can lead to potentially fatal complications such as cardiac arrhythmias, cardiovascular collapse and respiratory arrest.

- Early recognition of clinical signs of toxicity and their prompt treatment is vital.

Regional anaesthesia

The simplicity of administration of topical, infiltration and minor nerve-block anaesthesia has ensured its popularity for casualty work, dentistry and minor surgery. These techniques, along with epidural and spinal blockade, play a key role in both the prevention and treatment of pain and have much to offer patients, surgeons and anaesthetists (Table 1).

Local anaesthetics (LA) are the drugs most commonly used for regional techniques but other agents have been employed via the spinal and epidural route such as opioids, clonidine and the anaesthetic drug, ketamine. Before any regional technique is employed, it is worth remembering the important points summarized in Fig. 1 to minimise complications.

Regional anaesthesia is very versatile and can be used:

- Instead of general anaesthesia.
- As an adjuvant to general anaesthesia.
- With or without sedation.
- To relieve postoperative pain, e.g. epidural anaesthesia.

Regional techniques can be performed at a variety of sites throughout the body but the actual area affected depends on where the anaesthetic agent is introduced and the tissue targeted, e.g. single peripheral nerve or spinal cord. The choice of technique is also dependent upon the site of pain; the setting (out-patient clinic, operating theatre or ward) and the degree of expertise required to perform the task.

Single injection techniques can be useful for outpatient and minor surgical

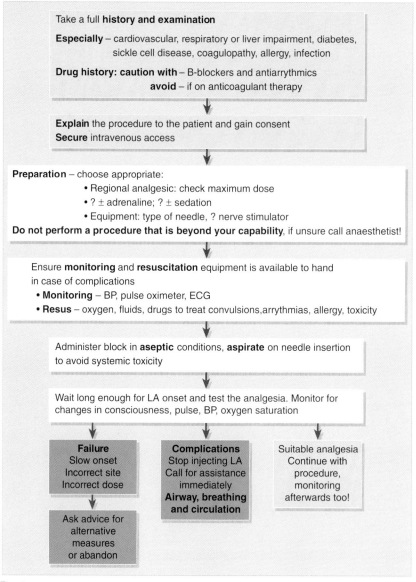

Take a full **history and examination**

Especially – cardiovascular, respiratory or liver impairment, diabetes, sickle cell disease, coagulopathy, allergy, infection

Drug history: caution with – B-blockers and antiarrythmics
avoid – if on anticoagulant therapy

Explain the procedure to the patient and gain consent
Secure intravenous access

Preparation – choose appropriate:
- Regional analgesic: check maximum dose
- ? ± adrenaline; ? ± sedation
- Equipment: type of needle, ? nerve stimulator

Do not perform a procedure that is beyond your capability, if unsure call anaesthetist!

Ensure **monitoring** and **resuscitation** equipment is available to hand in case of complications
- **Monitoring** – BP, pulse oximeter, ECG
- **Resus** – oxygen, fluids, drugs to treat convulsions, arrythmias, allergy, toxicity

Administer block in **aseptic** conditions, **aspirate** on needle insertion to avoid systemic toxicity

Wait long enough for LA onset and test the analgesia. Monitor for changes in consciousness, pulse, BP, oxygen saturation

Failure
Slow onset
Incorrect site
Incorrect dose

Complications
Stop injecting LA
Call for assistance immediately
Airway, breathing and circulation

Suitable analgesia
Continue with procedure, monitoring afterwards too!

Ask advice for alternative measures or abandon

Fig. 1 **Flow diagram to summarize the management of a patient undergoing regional analgesia.**

Table 1 **Benefits and contraindications of local infiltration and regional anaesthesia**		
GO **Benefits**	**THINK** **Cautions**	**STOP** **Contraindications**
Preservation of consciousness	Small children	Patient refusal
– Preservation of protective airway reflexes + reduced risk of aspiration	Cardiovascular disease	Not suitable as sole technique for certain operations
– Patient cooperation during the procedure	Beta-blocker/ anti-arrhythmic drugs	Poor cooperation
– Early detection of worsening medical condition, e.g. hypoglycaemia in diabetes, chest pain in angina	Liver impairment	Anticoagulation therapy
Limited effect on co-morbidity, e.g. COAD, angina		Bleeding disorder
Reduces the stress response to surgery		Infection
Improved postoperative outcome		Allergy
– Decreased incidence of DVT and PE		
Reduced intraoperative blood loss and transfusion requirements		
Provides optimal intraoperative and (in some cases) postoperative pain control		
– Reduced analgesic requirement		
– Reduced incidence/severity of opioid-induced side-effects		

procedures, while a continuous catheter technique may be preferred in the hospitalised patient who has under gone more extensive surgery.

Topical analgesia is covered on pages 88.

Local infiltration

LA is injected subcutaneously to anaesthetize the immediate surrounding area. Onset is within about 2 minutes and lasts from 30 minutes to 1 hour, depending on local circulation and dose. 1% and 2% lignocaine is routinely used, solutions either plain or with adrenaline. Adrenaline reduces blood loss and extends the duration of analgesia. Example of when to use: cleaning, exploration and suturing of wounds in A&E.

Field block

Field block involves subcutaneous infiltration around the operative field to produce a wall of analgesia. As the area involved with a field block can be quite large, relatively greater volumes of local anaesthetic are required. To avoid overdose, the maximum safe dose should be noted (with/without adrenaline) and using a precautionary low concentration of LA should be considered. Example of when to use: inguinal hernia repair.

Nerve block

These can be divided into proximal nerve blocks (e.g. brachial plexus) and peripheral nerve blocks (e.g. femoral nerve and ulnar nerve). The LA is injected into the tissue immediately next to the target nerve. Diffusion into the nerve will be slow and duration of analgesia longer in large nerves and vice versa for small nerves. For most nerve blocks 1% plain lignocaine with or without adrenaline is the most popular agent, although 0.5% bupivacaine is useful for prolonged analgesia.

Example of when to use: femoral nerve block for pain control of femoral fractures.

Intravenous regional anaesthesia

This technique (also known as 'Bier's block') exsanguinates the limb using a tourniquet, then injects a large dose of LA (30–40 ml of plain 0.5% prilocaine) into the venous system in the hand. Analgesia is established within 5–10 minutes. It is frequently used to provide anaesthesia for reduction of wrist fractures and minor surgery below the elbow. The tourniquet cuff must remain inflated for at least 20 minutes and be deflated slowly. If signs of toxicity are observed the tourniquet is re-inflated. This procedure must only be attempted by trained staff with resuscitation equipment readily available, due to relatively higher risk of systemic side-effects. Bier's block is contraindicated in patients with severe hypertension, peripheral vascular disease, obesity and sickle cell disease or trait. Example of when to use: reduction of Colles' fracture or minor surgery below the elbow.

Epidural anaesthesia

Epidural blocks can provide complete analgesia/anaesthesia to the thorax, abdomen or lower limbs. This technique is a suitable method for pain control in obstetrics, urology and some general abdomen and orthopaedic surgery. The LA can be administered either as a single dose or by top-ups via a catheter if prolongation of analgesia is desired.

Motor, sensory and autonomic blockade occurs following injection of LA into the epidural space. Hospitals have varying policies about where patients with epidurals in situ can be nursed, e.g. HDU only or on general wards. Ward staff must be specially trained and educated wherever epidurals are used and clear guidelines must be in place to manage any complications encountered. Epidural block height must be closely monitored, especially when continuous infusions of local anaesthetics are employed.

Example of when to use: gynaecological and urological surgery.

The side-effects or complications of epidural block may be classified as:

- An extended consequence of neural blockade (relatively common in occurrence).
- Technique-related (less common).

Complications arising from epidural blockade and their treatment are dealt with in more detail in 'Useful advice for house officers and non-anaesthetists' on pages 102–103.

Spinal anaesthesia

Spinal anaesthesia is performed by the injection of LA into the CSF in the subarachnoid space. Its use tends to be restricted to surgery below the level of the umbilicus and in obstetrics. The extent and duration of anaesthesia depends on factors affecting the spread of the LA agent. These include the position of the patient, the specific gravity of the LA, the level of injection (usually in the lumbar vertebral column), dose and volume of the agent.

This technique, like epidural analgesia, requires the expertise of an anaesthetist. Headache used to be a common problem post spinal puncture prior to the introduction of the atraumatic, pencil-point needles currently in use.

Example of when to use: major joint replacement (hip/knee), Caesarian sections and urology surgery.

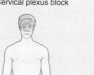

Fig. 2 **Possible regional techniques for pain management.**

Shoulder/arm/hand
- Brachial plexus block
- Local infiltration
- Bier's block
- Intra-articular injection
- Median/ulnar/radial nerve block
- Topical

Ano-genital
- Caudal
- Penile block
- Epidural/spinal
- Topical

Leg
- Femoral block
- Sciatic block
- Intra-articular
- Local infiltration
- Epidural/spinal
- Topical

Head and neck
- Infiltration
- Cervical plexus block

Chest
- Epidural
- Intercostal block
- Interpleural
- Paravertebral
- Topical

Abdomen
- Epidural
- Spinal
- Wound infiltration
- Inguinal field block
- Topical

Feet
- Ankle block
- Digital nerve block
- Local infiltration
- Topical

Regional anaesthesia

- Explain the procedure thoroughly to the patent and gain consent.
- Never attempt a procedure which is beyond your personal capability.
- Always check the maximum safe dose of the agent being used.
- Always aspirate on injection to avoid intravascular administration.
- Ensure resuscitation equipment is readily available.
- Monitor the patient for side-effects and toxicity during and after the procedure.
- If in doubt, or merely concerned, call for help.
- Complications can be serious.

Chronic pain syndromes

Chronic pain is a multidimensional problem that often leads to significant life disruption for patients and their families. Chronic pain is persistent and while often attributed to a physical cause, continues beyond the healing phase (usually accepted as 4–6 weeks).

Chronic pain can arise from many sources (Fig. 1). Some of the more common non-cancer conditions will be covered in this chapter. Cancer pain will be covered on pages 100–101.

Chronic low back pain

It is estimated that 80–90% of adults will experience an episode of back pain at some time during their lifetime, although the majority resolve within 2 weeks without specific treatment. Economically, chronic low back pain costs the NHS a total of £480 million/year, and in the UK it accounts for 11 million lost working days per year.

Management options for treatment of chronic low back pain include:

- Medication (NSAIDs, weak opioid drugs).
- Physiotherapy and exercise programmes.
- Psychology.
- Adjuvant therapies (e.g. TENS and acupuncture).
- Pain management programmes.
- Surgery (less common now)

Neuropathic pain

Neuropathic pain occurs as a consequence of sustained nerve damage and can arise from many different aetiologies, e.g. trauma, infection, metabolic disturbances, vascular insufficiency. To date, no drug has been developed exclusively for the treatment of neuropathic pain but tricyclic antidepressant drugs, anticonvulsant drugs and anti-arrhythmic drugs have all been used successfully.

The main types of neuropathic pain states are:

- Postoperative neuralgia.
- Postherpetic neuralgia.
- Trigeminal neuralgia
- Complex Regional Pain Syndrome.
- Phantom limb pain.

Postoperative neuralgia

Postoperative neuralgia (scar pain) is extremely difficult to manage because the aetiology of postoperative wound pain is frequently unknown. Pain may be a consequence of damage to bone, nerve or muscle, however the major component of scar pain is considered to be neuropathic in origin. This pain may be associated with numbness, pins and needles and abnormal temperature sensitivity.

Thoraco-abdominal incisions are particularly likely to result in postsurgical neuralgia, e.g. thoracotomy, inguinal hernia repair. The first-line management is pharmacological, using membrane-stabilizing agents such as anticonvulsants (valproate) or central nervous system-modifying drugs like the tricyclic antidepressants (amitriptyline). Pain control may be

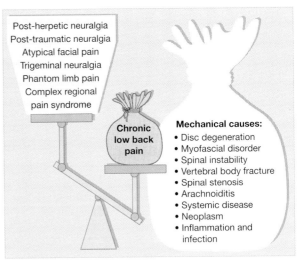

Fig. 1 **Chronic pain syndromes.**

achieved with injection of local anaesthetics and steroids. More permanent lesioning (e.g. cryotherapy) of the identified disruptive nerve can also be employed but has been found in some cases to make the pain worse.

Postherpetic neuralgia

Postherpetic neuralgia is caused by reactivation of the varicella zoster virus, which remains in latent form in the dorsal root ganglia following resolution of an acute herpetic infection (shingles). The precipitating factors for its reactivation are not understood, however on reactivation the virus replicates and transcends the sensory nerves to produce a papular rash over a dermatomal distribution, commonly the thoracic dermatomes and the ophthalmic division of the trigeminal nerve.

Postherpetic neuralgia:

- Follows an acute herpetic attack (shingles).
- Persists beyond 6 months (average duration 2 years).
- Increases in incidence with age (majority of patients referred to pain clinics are > 60 years).
- Gives burning or shooting pain aggravated by light touch.
- Causes problematic scarring and itching over the area.

Trigeminal neuralgia

This is a primary neuralgia usually of unknown aetiology, but can be associated with tumour, varicella zoster or multiple sclerosis. Trigeminal neuralgia can be confused with atypical facial pain (which does not follow a nerve distribution) and is often a diagnosis made on exclusion of other causes of facial pain, e.g. dental pain.

- Often unknown aetiology.
- Twice as common on the right side of the face.
- Middle-aged more affected.
- Ratio of women to men is 2:1.
- Pain is triggered by non-painful stimuli (allodynia) and results in hyperalgesic response.
- Pain is severe and sharp but brief (seconds).
- Often accompanied by facial muscle spasm.

Complex regional pain syndrome

This classification encompasses a wide group of chronic pain conditions. Two major subsets of complex regional pain syndrome (CRPS) have been described. A detailed summary of the clinical features of CRPS types I & II is beyond the scope of this book, however Fig. 2 illustrates some of the common symptoms, including oedema and shiny skin in the hands (Fig. 3).

CRPS type I (formerly reflex sympathetic dystrophy) This group is a complex disorder or group of disorders that may develop after major or trivial trauma with or without obvious nerve lesions. It also occurs after central nervous system lesions such as stroke or without cause.

CRPS type II (formerly causalgia) This occurs following nerve injury and is usually confined to a single nerve distribution.

Phantom limb pain

This is a poorly understood phenomena where post-amputation patients report a range of sensations (proprioception, temperature, pain) arising from the missing limb. Pain in the stump may occur early after surgery often as a consequence of complications (e.g. wound

infection/dehiscence), but chronic pain may develop in well-healed stumps and is often attributed to neuroma formation. Phantom limb pains have also been reported following mastectomy and gastrectomy.

Treatment of chronic pain

Multidisciplinary pain clinics

In order for pain management clinics to address the full needs of their patients a multidisciplinary approach must be taken. This usually includes an anaesthetist or consultant physician, pain nurse, physiotherapist, support group and clinical psychologist. Complete relief from chronic pain is often not possible. The psychologist plays a valuable role in helping patients understand their illness and in learning cognitive coping techniques and relaxation skills. Fig. 4 shows the treatment options used in managing chronic pain states.

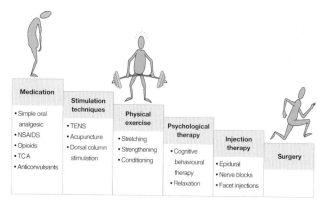

Fig. 4 **Treatment options in chronic pain management.**

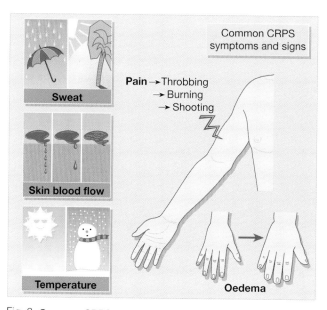

Fig. 2 **Common CRPS symptoms and signs.**

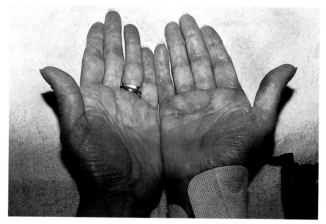

Fig. 3 **The shiny, oedematous skin of CRPS.**

> ### Clinical case 37
>
> You review a patient 12 weeks post Colle's fracture. The patient claims that the pain around her wrist is much worse than when she first broke it and that she has noticed a change in the appearance of the injured side. Her hand appears more swollen and shiny than the non-injured side and also feels cooler to touch. Her current medication is co-codamol tablets 3–4 per day.
>
> ■ What is the likely diagnosis?
> ■ What changes would you make to her current medication?
> ■ What other forms of treatment might be considered for her?
>
> *See comment on page 126.*

> ### Chronic pain syndromes
>
> ■ Chronic pain is common and often difficult to treat.
> ■ Chronic pain affects the patient physically, psychologically, socially and spiritually.
> ■ Relief from chronic pain is often transient and rarely complete.
> ■ Failure of treatment can precipitate fear, anger and a feeling of helplessness.
> ■ Anxiety can heighten the response to pain and fear of evoking pain can result, in avoidance of use, leading to a disuse syndrome.
> ■ For chronic pain to be managed effectively, a multidisciplinary approach should be employed.

Complementary medicine and analgesia

Complementary medicine embraces a wide range of therapeutic practices which at one time were considered as an alternative to mainstream Western practice. The mechanisms by which these various therapies work are not fully understood. However, interest in complementary medicine is growing and it is estimated that 10% of the UK public visit or have visited a complementary therapist. Many of the therapies are now offered within the NHS, usually (but not exclusively) as an adjuvant for pain relief.

Acupuncture

Acupuncture has been practiced in China for several thousand years and involves the insertion of tiny needles at specific points on the surface of the body (see Fig. 1). After insertion, the needles may be stimulated manually or by connecting them to a mild electrical current (electroacupuncture). According to ancient Chinese medical theory, the life force (Ch'i) flows through the body via 14 invisible channels (meridians), regulating all physical and mental processes.

Opposing forces within the body (yin and yang) must be balanced to keep ch'i flowing properly. The meridians run deep within the body's tissues and

Table 1 **Examples of conditions suitable for acupuncture analgesia**
Backache
Migraine and chronic headaches
Frozen shoulder and bursitis
Arthritis and gout
Repetitive strain injury
Carpal tunnel syndrome
Sports injury
Phantom limb pain
Chronic and terminal illness
Post-op. pain

organs, surfacing at some 360 places identified as acupuncture points (acupoints). Certain meridians are identified with organs (e.g. bladder, liver) and the points on the meridians are believed capable of affecting the associated internal organ. Stimulating these points is said to balance and restore the flow of ch'i.

The exact mechanism of action is still unknown, but it would appear that acupuncture stimulates myelinated A-delta fibres 'closing the gate' to higher centres from pain information conveyed in the small, unmyelinated C fibres. Acupuncture has also been demonstrated to increase the release of endogenous endorphins and alter the output of neurotransmitters such as serotonin and noradrenaline, blunting the perception of pain.

It is estimated that between 50–70% of patients with chronic pain receive at least temporary relief when treated with acupuncture (see Table 1).

Osteopathy and chiropractic

Osteopathy and chiropractic techniques are principally used in the treatment of acute and chronic back pain. It is proposed that by realigning the body through mobilizing joints and connective tissue, movement will be restored in restricted joints. Improved mobility should in turn lead to an improvement in general health. Traditionally, chiropractic techniques centre mainly around the affected joint, while osteopathy lays equal emphasis on the joint and adjacent muscles, ligaments and fascia.

One of the most common techniques used is a 'high velocity manipulation'.

This involves quick manipulation of a displaced area back into position with a very short joint movement. Chiropractic therapy is not recommended for disorders other than of musculoskeletal origin, and is best avoided where any of the following are present: osteoporosis, bone or joint infections, bone cancer, acute rheumatoid arthritis and diseases of the spinal cord or bone marrow. Serious side-effects from spinal manipulation appear to be rare (i.e. cerebrovascular event or stroke incidence of occurrence = 1/10 million manipulations).

Reflexology

Reflexology involves pressure and massage of various reflex points found on the feet and hands. The term 'reflex' is used in the sense of reflection, or mirror image, where tender areas on the feet and hands are thought to represent areas of imbalance elsewhere in the body (See Fig. 2). The right side of the body is reflected in the right foot, the left side in the left foot. Localized manipulation of these foot areas serves as treatment specific for disorders affecting the corresponding body areas. There have been no major clinical trials to verify the theories put forward for the mechanism of action of reflexology, but the theories outlined in Table 2 have been proposed.

Homeopathy

Homeopathic remedies are extremely diluted solutions (usually 1 part per million or less) of assorted herbs, animal products, and chemicals. They are so dilute that it's impossible to detect the original active ingredient in laboratory tests. Advocates of this therapy maintain

Fig. 1 **Patient with acupuncture needles in situ showing localized skin response.**

Table 2 **Proposed mechanisms of action for reflexology techniques**
■ Manipulation of the feet may reduce lactic acid in the tissues
■ Pressure on the reflex points may trigger the release of endorphins
■ Reflexology may induce a relaxation response, opening blood vessels and improving circulation
■ Manipulation may dissolve crystals of uric acid that settle in the feet, resulting in a detoxifying effect

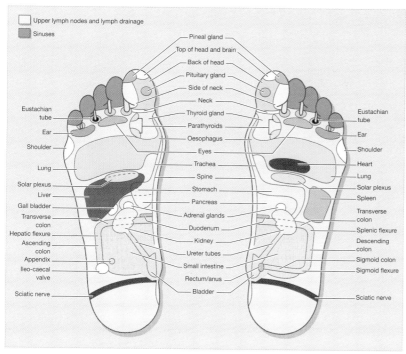

Fig. 2 **The reflexology map of human feet.**

that certain homeopathic medicines are more effective than a placebo in the treatment of certain conditions. It is proposed that the body is extremely sensitive to the homeopathic remedy and that these remedies stimulate the body into repairing itself. Again however, large randomized controlled clinical trials are lacking and there is no evidence for the mechanism of action of these remedies. Homeopathic medicines are available without a prescription. A homeopathic practitioner (who may be a physician, chiropractor, or unlicensed entrepreneur) typically begins by taking a lengthy medical history and then builds a 'symptom picture' against which to match homeopathy's extensive array of remedies.

Herbal medicine

Plants have been used for medical purposes for at least 5000 years and modern herbalism is probably the most common practiced form of medicine worldwide. Herbs are usually prescribed in combinations of between 2 and 12 (see Table 3). Despite little evidence for the mechanism of action of the various remedies used by herbalists, current theories include:

- Herbal medicines elicit a protective physiological response from the body.
- Herbs act as a food to supply the tissue with vital nutrients needed to regain normal cellular function.

- Herbs increase the detoxification of the body by enhancing the action of the organs of excretion.

It is estimated that up to 10–20% of people aged 18–25 years may take

Table 3 Examples of herbal remedies alleviating pain

Herbal medicine	Condition
Evening primrose oil	Breast pain
Capsicum cream	Arthritic pain and tenderness
Cranberry juice	Cystitis
Liquorice root	Stomach ulcer pain
Aloe vera	Inflammatory pain

Table 4 Summary of effects of cannabinoids

Analgesia	Appears similar to codeine
Anti-emetic	May be useful in chemotherapy patients
Sedation	Generalised CNS depression, drowsiness, dizziness, sleep
Cognition	Memory impairment, fragmentation of thoughts
Psychological	Euphoria, dysphoria, anxiety, hallucinations, paranoia, depression

cannabis weekly or more frequently. Cannabis belongs to the group of compounds known collectively as the cannabinoids. The cannabinoids are derived primarily from the female plant of *Cannabis sativa*. The most abundant cannabinoid and the main psychoactive constituent is d-9 tetrahydrocannabinol (THC). The THC content is highest in the flowering tops of the plant. Marijuana has a THC content of 0.5–5% and is prepared from the dried flowering tops and leaves. Hashish has a THC content somewhere between 2 and 20% and is composed of dried cannabis resin and compressed flowers. Cannabinoids have been reported to decrease the spasticity and pain associated with multiple sclerosis and spinal cord injuries. The analgesic efficacy of THC appears to be approximately equivalent to codeine. Nabilone is a commercially available cannabinoid used as an anti-emetic in anticancer treatment. It is usually given in a dose of 4–8 mg per day in divided doses during chemotherapy. However, 50–100% of patients experience drowsiness, dizziness and lethargy while taking it. It is obvious that more controlled studies must be performed before the place of these compounds in clinical practice can be fully determined, and indeed much research is currently on-going. It is highly likely that the psychotropic side-effects associated with current agents would limit their role to that of an adjuvant rather than a first line therapy in pain management.

Complementary medicine and analgesia

- Complementary medicine constitutes a huge and rapidly growing industry.
- Complementary therapies are increasingly being incorporated into pain management.
- It is advisable to consult a doctor before visiting a complementary therapist if symptoms are new, persistent or worsening.
- Complementary medicine works alongside traditional medicine and should not be seen as an alternative to regular medical care.
- Professional training is required to gain competency in these fields so it is wise to refer only to members of a professionally recognized organization.

ABCDs of pain management problems

Pain in AIDS, burns, crisis of sickle cell, drug addicts (ABCDs)

There are certain conditions where pain is often poorly treated despite being a significant symptom. These pages focus on pain management in four such conditions.

Analgesia in AIDS patients

The unpredictability of disease progression in AIDS patients makes pain management and palliative care problematic. Pain problems are common in HIV disease, affecting at least 60% in terminal stages. Pain has a huge impact on quality of life and is a significant risk factor for depression and suicide.

Effective pain management requires diagnosis. Nociceptive, neuropathic and idiopathic pains are all commonly seen in AIDS patients. While nociceptive pain may respond to NSAIDs and opiates; neuropathic pain, a common complaint of HIV, may be more difficult to relieve (see 'Acute pain management' on pages 84–85).

See Fig. 1 for specific pain problems in AIDS patients.

Treatment goals

Treat primary pathology with specific agents where possible, e.g. acyclovir for herpes zoster outbreaks (occurs in 5–10% of HIV-positive patients). Symptomatic treatment of pain should be started as soon as possible, incorporating step-ups along the analgesic ladder (see 'Cancer Pain Management' on page 100). Consider using prophylactic agents, e.g. H_2 blockers in oesophageal disease and topical lignocaine gel in rectal/anal pain. Colic and visceral pains can be opioid responsive but may need anticholinergic adjuvants, e.g. hyoscine.

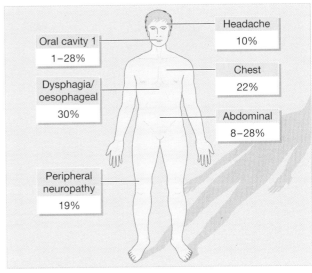

Fig. 1 **Pain symptoms in AIDS patients.**

Analgesia in burns patients

Not all burn injuries are painful! Some burns are extremely painful whereas others are pain-free:

- Superficial (first-degree) burns (Fig. 2) – sensory nerve endings are intact, therefore painful.
- Partial thickness (second-degree) burns – sensory nerve endings are intact, therefore painful.
- Full-thickness (third-degree) burns – sensory nerve endings are destroyed, therefore pain-free.

Frequently burn injuries are extremely painful and unfortunately analgesia is often under-prescribed and under-administered as the efforts of the clinicians are focused on the diagnosis and treatment of the life-threatening complications of the burns.

Opiates are the most widely used form of analgesia in severe burns patients. Intravenous administration is the route of choice; if given subcutaneously or intramuscularly in the recently burned patient, the morphine may remain unabsorbed until the circulation improves (possibly several hours later). This could give rise to unexpected respiratory depression and loss of consciousness.

Optimal relief of burn pain may require adjuvant treatments to opiates (see Table 1).

Ongoing psychological support is absolutely essential as the burn injury not only gives rise to short-term changes and severe pain, but to chronic pain and perhaps permanent disfigurement. Relaxation, imagery and biofeedback can be incorporated into the patient's treatment to maximize management pain.

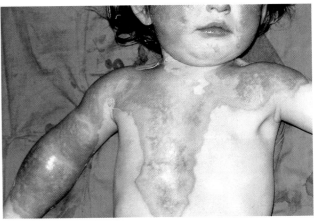

Fig. 2 **Painful superficial burn in a young child** (reproduced courtesy of Mr JD Holmes, Consultant Plastic Surgeon, Aberdeen Royal Infirmary).

Table 1 Adjuvant treatments to opiates for optimal pain-relief in burns

Analgesia for changing dressings can be self or nurse-administrated, e.g. Entonox

Simple analgesics (paracetamol/aspirin) can relieve some of the discomfort of a burn wound that may otherwise keep the patient restless with sleepless nights. If the pain is more severe consider dihydrocodeine or pentazocine

Antidepressants appear to enhance opiate-induced analgesia

TENS, psychological techniques and local anaesthetics are also useful

In severe cases continuous sedation may be required (in HDU or ICU setting)

Pain in sickle cell disease (SCD)

Pain is the most common manifestation of SCD after the age of 2 years and painful episodes are most frequent from 20–40 years-of-age. Most patients with SCD are managed in the community by their GP and painful episodes self-managed at home with oral analgesia and fluids. However, it is important for the house officer to be able to treat appropriately the patient presenting in A&E with an acute painful crisis.

The acute pain crisis of SCD results from microvascular occlusion, caused by the cumulative effects of haemoglobin S (HbS) polymerization, red cell sickling, sickle cell adhesion to vascular endothelium and fibrin deposition. The severity and location of the acute pain arising from an infarctive crisis may vary and the crisis duration may last from a few minutes to several weeks.

Precipitating factors of acute pain in SCD
- Cold.
- Dehydration.
- Alcohol.
- Stress.
- Concurrent infection.
- Menstruation.

In more than 50% of cases no precipitant cause can be identified.

Management of the painful crisis in SCD
The acute pain team should be involved as early as possible and most hospitals who deal frequently with sickle cell patients will have an established protocol for triage and pain management (see Table 2). A minority of patients suffer from severe pain almost constantly. Recurrent episodes of vaso-occlusion and infarction may lead to chronic neuropathic-type pain developing. Management of chronic pain requires expert advice.

Intravenous drug abuse and pain

When patients with a history of substance abuse present with severe pain, they are often viewed by caregivers as already having had too much opioid and only seeking to support their habit. This may result in withholding opioids from such patients and precipitate withdrawal symptoms.

Users withdrawing from opiates may experience:
- Nausea, vomiting and diarrhoea.
- Insomnia, agitation and restlessness.
- Muscle, bone and joint pain.
- Gooseflesh ('cold turkey') and flushing.
- Abdominal cramps.
- Dilated pupils.

Acute pain with a clear origin (e.g. post-traumatic postoperative) nearly always warrants treatment with a strong opioid, albeit on a short-term basis. It is important to be aware of the need for such pain-relief in heroin users.

Non-opiate treatment regimens should also be incorporated, such as:

Neuroleptic drugs, e.g. phenothiazines with their anti-emetic, sedative and anticholinergic effects. The latter help to reduce abdominal cramps, which can be a distressing symptom of opiate withdrawal.

Antispasmodics, (e.g. mebeverine) used to relieve colicky abdominal pain.

Simple analgesics, (e.g. paracetamol) may be sufficient to relieve muscular aches and pains.

Methadone, given orally as a substitute drug is also an accepted part of the management of intravenous opiate users. Its use can reduce/prevent withdrawal symptoms and eliminates the risk of injection and needle-sharing, enabling the patient to stabilise drug intake and lifestyle.

Table 2 Sickle cell pain management.

Acute severe painful episodes	Chronic pain	Prevention of pain crisis
Opiates should be given at frequent and fixed intervals, e.g. PCA iv morphine 1 mg bolus, 5 minute lockout	Fentanyl patches or oral morphine preparations for prolonged moderate to severe pain	Lifestyle – avoid alcohol and resultant dehydration
Consider adjuvant analgesics, e.g. NSAIDs	Paracetamol with codeine for mild to moderate pain	Hydroxyurea – an attempt to increase the production of HbF, inhibiting HbS polymerization
Treat nausea if present, e.g. prochlorperazine	NSAIDs for bone pain	
Give supplementary oxygen		
Don't forget to replace fluids liberally!		
Don't forget to treat the cause!		

ABCDs of pain management problems
- It is important to be aware of the significant distress pain can cause in common medical conditions and to have a basic understanding of the various treatment options.
- A better understanding of the aetiology of the pain will help to effectively treat it.
- Opioids are the treatment of choice in the acute painful crisis (e.g. of SCD, major burns).
- Nociceptive, neuropathic and idiopathic pains are all commonly seen in HIV/AIDS patients and require different approaches to treatment, often incorporating the chronic pain physicians.

Pain in the young and the old

Until recently, it was widely held that the human neonate was not capable of perceiving pain. Current research suggests that the opposite is true: in the human foetus, pain pathways are well developed in late gestation, and the neurochemical systems associated with pain transmission and modulation are intact and functional (Fig. 1).

The use of sedation, analgesia, local and general anaesthesia during painful procedures in neonates and young infants should be applied as they are to children and adults in similar situations.

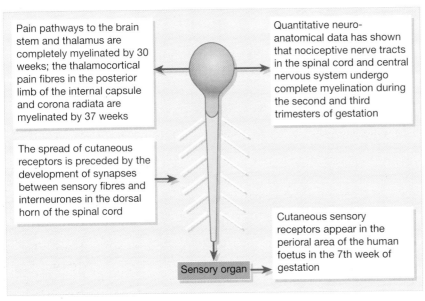

Pain pathways to the brain stem and thalamus are completely myelinated by 30 weeks; the thalamocortical pain fibres in the posterior limb of the internal capsule and corona radiata are myelinated by 37 weeks

The spread of cutaneous receptors is preceded by the development of synapses between sensory fibres and interneurones in the dorsal horn of the spinal cord

Quantitative neuro-anatomical data has shown that nociceptive nerve tracts in the spinal cord and central nervous system undergo complete myelination during the second and third trimesters of gestation

Cutaneous sensory receptors appear in the perioral area of the human foetus in the 7th week of gestation

Sensory organ

Fig. 1 **Development of nociception in the foetus.**

Table 1 Methods of pain assessment in young children

Form of assessment	Self-report tools	Concept of order observation	Behavioural	Physiological measures
Age of Patient	Most children ≥ 4 years	≥ 7 years	Preverbal and nonverbal children	All
Method	Various (e.g. faces scale)	Numerical or word-graphic rating scale	Vocalizations, facial expressions, motor responses, posture	Heart rate Blood pressure
Use	Primary	Primary	Adjuvant	Adjuvant
Accuracy	✓✓✓	✓✓	✓	✗

Table 2 Routes of administration of analgesia in children

Route	Age-range	Risk of intoxication	Continuous concentration present	Restricts movement	Other
PCA	≥ 5 years	Increased	✓✓	✓✓	Sedation
Morphine infusion	All	Much increased	✓✓✓	✓✓	Close nursing
Epidural infusion	All	Increased	✓✓	✓	Eliminates injections Less sedating, fewer or no opioid side-effects
Regional or nerve block	All	Much decreased	✓	✓	Prevents wind-up, opioid-sparing effect

PAIN MEASUREMENT SCALE

NO PAIN	COMFORTABLE EXCEPT ON MOVING	PERSISTENT DISCOMFORT	DISTRESSING PAIN	UNBEARABLE PAIN
0	1	2	3	4

GRASEBY

Fig. 2 **Faces pain-rating scale.**

Pain management in children

Despite effective techniques, pain in children is often managed less well than in adults. Early management is crucial, as once established severe pain can be difficult to control.

Before drugs are used in the treatment of pain, non-pharmacological interventions such as parental presence, pacifiers, familiar toys and touch (i.e. swaddling, stroking, rocking, caressing, massaging, and cuddling) should be tried.

The pharmacological treatment chosen depends on the child's age, medical condition, type of surgery and expected postoperative course. NSAIDs are often used first-line or in combination with opioids. Special considerations are given to premature infants, neonates and children with neurological abnormalities or pulmonary diseases, as they are more susceptible to apnoea and respiratory depression with the use of systemic opioids.

Pain evaluation in children is difficult and is often the reason for pain being undertreated. Difficulty exists in younger children in distinguishing between anxiety and pain. Despite the availability and relative simplicity of pain-assessment tools for children (see Table 1 and Fig. 2), formal assessments are still not widely performed.

Dosing and administration

Practical points to remember for administering analgesia in children:

Avoid the intramuscular route where possible: use oral, rectal (obtain consent from child/parent) and intravenous routes first.

Titrate the opioid (dose and interval) until desired analgesic effect is achieved.

Offer rescue doses for breakthrough or poorly controlled pain.

Reduce the initial dose and monitor infants < 6 months-of-age.

The intravenous route can be used for bolus administration and continuous infusion, including PCA where child-friendly handset can be employed (Fig. 3).

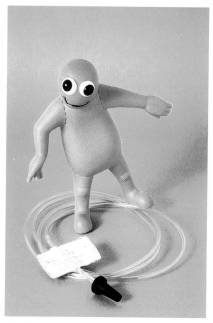

Fig. 3 **Child-friendly hand piece.**

Pain in the elderly

The incidence of pain in people over 60 is twice that of people under 60, with 25–50% of the elderly population experiencing pain problems.

Cancer, musculoskeletal disease and vascular disease are some of the conditions responsible for the incidence of pain in older people. Other causes are shown in Fig. 4. Multiple illness and pathology make the picture more complex, as well as chronic illnesses being more common, e.g. arthritis. Increasing age and complex medication regimens place the elderly population at increased risk for drug–drug and drug–disease interactions.

Pain behaviour and assessment

Reasons why the elderly may be less likely to report their pain include the following:

- Fear of 'bothering' or 'annoying' those responsible for their care.
- Inability to report clearly, because of speech, hearing, cognitive deficits or language barriers (see 'The elderly' on pages 36 and 37).
- Fear of facing pain, because it could lead to more serious illness or even death.
- Concerns about drug therapy and limitations to 'mix medications'.
- Belief that pain has to be endured because of the ageing process.

A detailed pain assessment should be performed including evaluation of psychological and social function.

Formal pain assessments may not be possible for those with speech, hearing or cognitive deficits or who fear reporting pain. For visual, hearing, motor, and cognitive impairments the use of simple descriptive, numeric, and visual analogue pain-assessment instruments may be impeded, and cognitively impaired patients may require simpler scales and more frequent pain assessment.

Physiological, psychological and anatomical changes in the elderly must be considered when prescribing analgesia. These changes are described in detail in 'The elderly' on pages 36 and 37. In addition, remember to incorporate the following points:

- Simplify prescribing where possible (e.g. slow-release preparations mean fewer tablets).
- Reduce dosage – start at 50% of normal adult dose.
- Minimize polypharmacy.
- Review regularly – to stop or reduce.

Not all drugs are bad but remember when treating elderly patients:

NSAID side-effects – higher incidence of gastric and renal toxicity and other drug reactions such as cognitive impairment, constipation, and headaches in older patients.

Opioid effectiveness – the elderly tend to be more sensitive to the analgesic and CNS-depressant effects of opioids.

Patient-controlled analgesia – slower drug clearance and increased sensitivity to undesirable drug effects (e.g. cognitive impairment) indicate the need for cautious initial dosing and subsequent titration and monitoring.

Clinical case 38

A distressed 74-year-old man is admitted as an emergency to your surgical ward. He has a painful ischaemic left lower leg with no pulses palpable below the knee and a gangrenous forefoot. A below-knee amputation will be necessary. He also gets pain in his other limb and occasional chest pain when he walks a short distance or gets upset. He has smoked 40 cigarettes a day for the past 60 years but despite having a chronic cough and wheeze, is unwilling to stop smoking. He lives alone with no family close-by, but attends a social club three times a week relying on public transport to do so. What factors may be contributing to his distress? What would the best option be to manage his pain? What preoperative risk-factors have been identified? What potential long-term problems might he experience as a consequence of his medical history?
See comment on page 126.

Pain in the young and the old

- Difficulty in evaluating pain means pain in the young and elderly can be under-treated.

- The use of standard pain-assessment tools in this group may be difficult. Use modified scales where possible, e.g. Oucher face scale, Activities of Daily Living score.

- A multimodal approach to analgesia should be used incorporating non-pharmacological approaches where possible.

- Utilize the oral route as much as possible.

- Be aware of age-related changes in drug pharmacodynamics and pharmacokinetics and adjust medication accordingly.

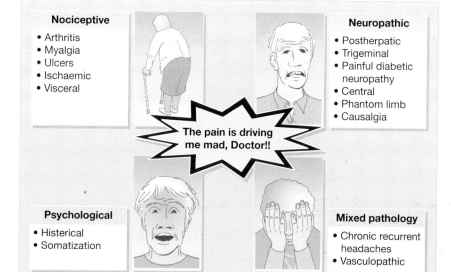

Nociceptive
- Arthritis
- Myalgia
- Ulcers
- Ischaemic
- Visceral

Neuropathic
- Postherpatic
- Trigeminal
- Painful diabetic neuropathy
- Central
- Phantom limb
- Causalgia

The pain is driving me mad, Doctor!!

Psychological
- Histerical
- Somatization

Mixed pathology
- Chronic recurrent headaches
- Vasculopathic

Fig. 4 **Causes of pain in the elderly.**

Cancer pain management

Around two-thirds of cancer patients experience pain as a symptom, often having more than one type of pain at any given time. In advanced cancer states, pain is present in up to 90% patients. Pain in cancer patients may be due to:

- Cancer itself (e.g. bone-marrow infiltration).
- Cancer treatment (e.g. chemotherapy mucositis).
- Cancer-induced debility (e.g. pressure sores).
- Unrelated disorder (e.g. osteoarthritis).

Assessment of cancer pain should follow the guidelines set out in Pain assessment on pages 78–79. Multimodal treatment is often required for cancer patients and their pain. Treatment should be directed at modifying the source of the pain with antineoplastic therapies, such as chemotherapy, radiotherapy and hormonal manipulation. Radiotherapy is often very effective for bone pain.

It may be that the patient's suffering has a spiritual or emotional component, e.g. a fear of dying, a sense of hopelessness. It is vital that these issues are identified and addressed within the pain-management strategy. Family and friends are important and should be involved where possible. Local hospice/hospital support team/home-care services should be considered. Good symptomatic pain relief maximizes the quality of the limited time available.

Pharmacotherapy

Pharmacological management is considered the first line of therapy for patients with cancer pain. The World Health Organization (WHO) introduced a step-like ladder as a guide to analgesia prescribing in cancer patients (Fig. 1).

The WHO ladder relies exclusively on oral administration and is usually effective. Between 70–90% of patients can be rendered relatively pain-free when its principles are applied in a thorough and careful manner. The mainstay of treatment cancer pain of moderate to severe intensity is with potent opioid analgesics (group III). Most patients will require simultaneous treatment with two different formulations of an opioid: a long-acting preparation administered by the clock and a short-acting, fast-onset analgesic given as required.

Morphine remains the standard reference to which other analgesics are compared and basal analgesia is usually provided by controlled release preparations of oral morphine every 8 or 12 hours, e.g. MST. Daily doses of morphine required to adequately relieve cancer pain may vary from 60–3000 mg in divided doses. Individuals vary in their sensitivity to the analgesic effects and toxicity of morphine.

Where side-effects with morphine are limiting its clinical usefulness, alternatives such as methadone, oxycodone, hydromorphone and transdermal fentanyl patches can be used. In addition to these long-acting preparations, potent short-acting opioids with minimal potential for accumulation may be required for breakthrough pain. When frequent breakthrough doses are required, the dose of the basal analgesic should be increased accordingly.

Route of administration

Treatment with potent opioid analgesics may be started in a variety of ways (Fig. 2). Independent of the route, it is preferable to commence with low starting doses and allow rapid upward titration. This allows a steady-state plasma level to be achieved, providing analgesia while limiting the frequency of side-effects, and enhances compliance. For patients requiring strong opioids long term, the non-invasive routes e.g. oral, transdermal, transmuscosal are preferred to parenteral administration. Most commonly, patients are titrated with an oral immediate-release formulation, which allows rapid onset but has a short duration of action.

Patients should start on a low dose which can be gradually increased as required. Starting doses of 5–10 mg oral morphine, at four hourly intervals, are suitable for most adults although this dose may have to be reduced in the elderly and if evidence of renal impairment is present. Once an effective daily dose has been achieved, a controlled-release formulation may be commenced.

The intravenous or subcutaneous route may be used where rapid control of severe pain is required, and later converted to an oral drug regimen. When using morphine this necessitates using a ratio of 1:3 (morphine sulphate 10 mg s.c. = 30 mg p.o.). Non-invasive routes should be maintained for as long as possible for simplicity, maintenance of independence, convenience and cost.

One-third to two-thirds of patients may benefit from at least the transient use of an alternative route sometime before death. Morphine can also be given by rectal administration for a short period for time if indicated. Other methods of administering opioids in advanced disease include the epidural and intrathecal routes.

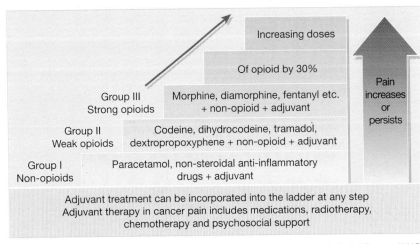

Fig. 1 **Analgesic ladder** (adapted from World Health Organization. Cancer Pain Relief. Geneve, WHO, 1986).

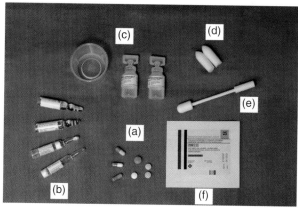

Fig. 2 **Opioid analgesics,** (a) Oral tablets/capsules, (b) parenteral IV/SC/IM, (c) oral solution, (d) rectal, (e) oral transmucosal (f) transdermal.

There is no evidence to suggest that parenteral analgesia produces superior analgesia to the oral route, so it should be reserved for patients incapable of oral ingestion or where high oral doses require an impractical number of tablets or produce unacceptable side-effects.

Opioid side-effects and their management

Long-term administration of potent opioids in cancer patient can produce side-effects, which are listed on page 83. Constipation and miosis are the only two opioid side-effects to which tolerance appears never to significantly develop. Constipation is almost invariable and prophylactic laxatives should be employed. Clinicians should be on the lookout for evidence of bowel obstruction and faecal impaction in these patients and treat promptly. Opioid-mediated nausea and sedation occur in up to half of patients first exposed to an opioid. These symptoms usually resolve spontaneously with continued use

Tolerance, physical dependency and addiction

Once these three conditions were considered together as part of a single syndrome, but now they are rightly recognized as three distinct phenomena. Physical dependency refers to the probability that a state of withdrawal will be experienced following abstinence from that drug. Tolerance occurs when over time an increased dose of the drug is required to produce the same effect. By using the oral route,

tolerance to opioids develops more slowly (and painful injections are avoided!). Addiction happens when there is an overwhelming desire to acquire a drug for non-medical use and use continues despite the presence or threat of physiological or psychological harm. Physical dependence and tolerance are invariably associated with chronic opioid use, but addiction is a rare sequelae of medical prescribing in cancer patients.

Invasive and procedural approches

For the 10–30% of patients whose pain remains refractory to the WHO analgesic ladder, invasive pain interventions may be of some help (see Table 1). Such treatments involve greater acute risk, often more demanding maintenance for families and carers and the specialist skills of usually either an anaesthetist or neurosurgeon.

Palliative care

It should be remembered that pain is only one of many symptoms that may need managed in patients with advanced cancer (Table 2). Multidisciplinary palliative care teams have been set up to ensure that cancer sufferers and their families achieve as much relief from these symptoms as possible. The hospice can provide a transition phase between hospital care and home, providing the patient with a strong support network to enable ongoing care in the community rather than a busy acute hospital ward.

Table 1 **Invasive procedures for cancer pain**		
Procedure	**Indication**	**Example**
Local anaesthetic blocks with local anaesthetic and corticosteroid	Fractured rib/pain from bony rib metastasis	Intercostal nerve blocks
Neurolytic blocks with alcohol or phenol	Abdominal pain	Coeliac plexus block
Neuroablative surgery	Localized refractory pain	Percutaneous cordotomy
Neuroaugmentative analgesics	Widespread, diffuse refractory lower-body pain	Epidural or intrathecal catheter with injection port or implanted pump

Table 2 **Frequency of symptoms in advanced cancer**	
Symptoms	**%**
Pain	70
Anorexia	50–90
Insomnia	20–80
Weakness	70
Immobility	85
Dry mouth	20–50
Constipation	40–50
Nausea	30–50
Vomiting	30–50
Dyspnoea	30–70
Oedema	30–40
Cough	30–75
Pressure sores	15–60
Incontinence	20–30
Psychological morbidity	25

Cancer pain management

- Cancer pain is multifactorial and dynamic, requiring continuous and consistent assessment.

- Cancer patients often have more than one pain at any given time.

- Not all pain in cancer is due to malignancy.

- Some pains, however intense, do not respond to morphine.

- Utilize the 'Rule of Fives' when prescribing analgesia:
  - By the mouth
  - By the clock
  - By the ladder
  - For the individual
  - Adding adjuvant medication.

Useful advice to house officers and non-anaestheists

All analgesic techniques have the potential to cause complications. An understanding of the drugs and techniques involved along with an ability to recognise and, if necessary, treat complications is essential for patient safety. The aim of this chapter is to highlight some of the problems that may occur on the ward when more complex (but frequently employed) techniques are used. Readers should re-read the chapters on postoperative complications. The main problems encountered from an analgesic modality can be divided into two main categories.

Drug-related analgesic problem areas

- Inadequate analgesia, e.g. inappropriate dosage, inappropriate drug used.
- Unacceptable side-effects, e.g. nausea/vomiting, sedation, respiratory depression.

Technique-related analgesic problem areas

- Equipment failure, e.g. PCA – programming errors (see Table 1).
- Failure of block technique.
- Significant neural blockade secondary to regional block.
- Complication specific to block technique.

Block failure

The success of regional anaesthesia depends on accurate placement of local anaesthetic solution in close proximity to nerve trunks. In most peripheral somatic nerve blocks, this depends upon paraesthesia being elicited by the doctor and reported by the patient. Success of the block may be poor due to inappropriate responses from the patient, perhaps as a result of apprehension, over-sedation or disorientation. To reduce this potential for error, the needle-tip can be located by mechanical aids such as a peripheral nerve stimulator, or in more invasive blocks such as coeliac plexus block by using fluroscopy.

Successful regional analgesia requires more than just technical skill in performing the nerve blocks themselves, preoperative, intraoperative and postoperative factors must be considered (Table 2).

Excessive blockade

Watch out for this on the ward! One of the more common side-effects of epidural blockade is hypotension caused by vasodilation from a sympathetic block. Sympathetic blockade may be a significant factor but true hypovolaemia is common after both major abdominal and thoracic surgery. Patients may have both absolute hypovolaemia due to inadequate fluid replacement and relative hypovolaemia due to sympathetic blockade. The reported incidence of hypotension associated with epidural bupivacaine varies much, from 0–60%. The severity of hypotension depends on the height of the block and the patients ability to compensate, making elderly patients and patients on beta-blockers particularly vulnerable. Hypotension is reported more frequently with thoracic than with lumbar epidurals. If the block extends up to T1–T4 a pronounced bradycardia due to sympathetic blockade of the cardio-accelerator fibres may also occur. Urinary retention may be masked as patients are unable to sense when their bladder is full.

These complications are usually transient, only lasting as long as the block is maintained, and mild enough not to require treatment. However, if severe or causing the patient discomfort, measures should be taken to treat the problem.

Hypotension can be managed by:

- administering oxygen
- postural adjustment
- sympathomimetic agents (e.g. ephedrine, adrenaline)

Table 2 **Preoperative, intraoperative and postoperative considerations when performing nerve blocks.**

Preoperative	Intraoperative	Postoperative
Explain procedure to patient in terms they understand and ensure full cooperation	Test the block If patient unsedated their cooperation is valuable Monitor pulse and BP	A motor block may result in: Problems walking Risk of falling/injury
Select appropriate premedications (if required), e.g. diazepam for anxiety	Treat a fall in BP > 30%: Give O_2 and fluids Raise legs Adrenaline/ephedrine If BP remains low, suspect occult haemorrhage!	Autonomic block: Hypotension Unable to micturate Bradycardia
Measure pulse and BP Secure iv access Give O_2 and fluids as required Empty bladder prior to analgesic block Major blocks: Nil by mouth on day of procedure	High spinals can cause decrease in inspiratory capacity Give ventilatory support If bladder over-distended a urinary catheter is required	Reduction in pain awareness may mask: Accidental injury Compartment syndrome Need to pass urine Possible causes of abnormal neurological sequelae: Haematoma Abscess Direct trauma

Table 1 **Drug-related problems encountered with a PCA device**

Inadequate analgesia	Respiratory depression	Nausea
At the start: Give a loading dose until patient comfortable then commence PCA programme	Stimulate the patient and titrate intravenous NALOXONE (opioid antagonist) to desired effect	Give an anti-emetic, e.g. prochlorperazine 12.5 mg im/pr
With few demands: Encourage the patient to use the PCA more frequently	Once resolved consider reducing bolus size and/or increasing the lockout period **Over-sedation**	Consider changing route of PCA, e.g. from iv to sc
With frequent demands: Check correct drug concentration, programme settings and patient connections Increase bolus size if no error in the above found	Treat as for respiratory depression	Consider changing to a different opioid, e.g. from morphine to fentanyl.

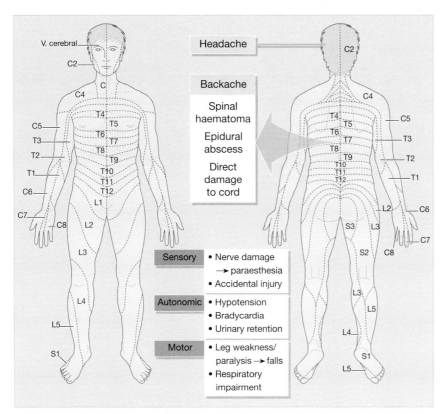

Fig. 1 **Complications of epidural blockade.**

Direct trauma to the spinal cord (lower risk below the 2nd lumbar vertebrae).

Epidural abscess is rare but more likely in immunocompromised patients or patients on steroids. An abscess may present as pain and neurological changes several days after epidural insertion and may be associated with localized tenderness, fever and leucocytosis. MRI is the best diagnostic tool and early surgical intervention is advised.

Urine retention can be relieved by bladder catheterization and the staff caring for the patient postoperatively should be vigilant for any deterioration in condition otherwise masked by the block.

The degree of lower-limb motor block appears to be related to the mass of local anaesthetic given and the site of the epidural catheter (greater for lumbar than thoracic sites).

Technique-related complications
Dural puncture may give rise to post-dural puncture headache (PDPH) resulting from cerebrospinal leakage and decreased intracranial pressure. The pain of PDPH is usually frontal but traction on the infratentorial structures can give rise to occipital and neck pain too. The rate of inadvertent dural puncture during epidural insertion is 0.6–1.3%. The likelihood of developing a PDPH varies between 16 and 86% as multiple factors are involved (Table 3).

Inadvertent spinal blockade (from LA entering the subarachnoid, resulting in an unintentional widespread block)

can result in paralysis of upper limbs and muscles of respiration such as the diaphragm and intercostal muscles, leading to respiratory impairment and hypoxia.

Puncture of an epidural vein may lead occasionally to a haematoma forming. Its occurrence is usually associated with a pre-existing coagulopathy. However, the risk of epidural haematoma may also be increased by concurrent use of prophylactic low-dose heparin or low molecular weight heparin. To minimize this risk, epidural catheters should ideally be removed 10–12 hours after the last heparin dose, and the anticoagulation should not be reinstituted for at least 2 hours after catheter removal.

Table 3 **Factors Increasing likelihood of PDPH**

Age in 2nd + 3rd decades
Female gender
Pregnancy
Dehydration
History of previous PDPH
Large needle gauge
Cutting bevel

Clinical case 39
A patient returns to the ward post-laparotomy, with an epidural catheter in situ. An injection (known as a top-up) of 10 ml of 0.25% plain bupivacaine was given by the anaesthetist 40 minutes earlier and a continuous infusion of 0.125% bupivacaine and 1 µg/ml fentanyl was started on return to the ward, running as prescribed at 8 ml/hour. The patient is concerned that something is wrong because he is having difficulty moving his legs and the nurse reports that his blood pressure is reading 85/40 mmHg. What explanation would you give the patient? How would you assess the extent of the patient's block? What instructions would you give the nurse looking after the patient?
See comment on page 126.

Advice to house officers and non-anaestheists

- All analgesic techniques have the potential to cause complications.
- As the complexity of the technique increases, so does the potential for harm.
- Complications can be drug-related or technique-related.
- Monitoring by trained staff is mandatory to recognize complications early before damage to the patient is inevitable.
- Communication is particularly important when advanced techniques are used. Seek help early as delaying appropriate treatment can seriously affect patient outcome.

What is intensive care?

The intensive care unit (ICU) is a designated area for management of the critically ill patient at a level that cannot be maintained elsewhere in the hospital. The ICU represents one end of a spectrum of care that begins in the community and outpatient departments, progresses to general wards and then to an intermediate level of care provided by the high-dependency unit (HDU).

High-dependency and intensive care facilities have a higher nurse to patient ratio than the normal wards and better access to specialist equipment (see Fig. 1). Staff members receive specialized training to work in intensive care and include doctors, nurses, physiotherapists, pharmacists, technicians and dieticians. Optimal patient care is achieved through close interaction between the admitting team and the intensive care multidisciplinary team (Figs. 2 & 3).

Early involvement of the ICU/HDU team is advisable to facilitate optimal care and timely transfer to intensive care should it become necessary. ICUs offer a variety of treatments for patients with multiple organ failure, regardless of the original disease. In addition the ICU offers care to patients prior to elective and emergency surgery, after major surgery (cardiothoracic, neurological, vascular, orthopaedic and abdominal) and to those patients following polytrauma, cardiorespiratory arrest and medical emergencies.

Criteria for admission

The ICU caters for patients with many conditions. The primary aim is to treat acute disturbances of organ function and physiology, so as to preserve life while the underlying pathology is diagnosed and treated. Patients can be admitted to the ICU for a number of reasons, but as a rule patients require the support of two or more organ systems, with support of single-organ systems being provided in the HDU environment. Patients with co-existing diseases, however, may require intensive care even if only one organ system is failing.

Generally speaking, advanced respiratory support (endotracheal intubation and/or mechanical ventilation) is also an indication for intensive care. Less invasive respiratory support, including continuous positive airway pressure (CPAP) and non-invasive ventilation, is usually safely instituted in an HDU.

Cost–benefit analysis

A stipulation for a patient's eligibility for admission to an ICU/HDU is that the acute deterioration should be considered reversible. Sadly, some patients are admitted to the ICU when there is no hope of recovery. This results in futile investigations, unnecessary suffering and loss of dignity, and merely delays the dying process. Decisions regarding ICU admission, as with cardiopulmonary resuscitation, should be considered an integral part of a patient's care.

ICU and HDU beds are expensive and finite resources, necessitating appropriate allocation. When a terminally ill patient occupies an ICU bed, a patient with a severe acute insult may be denied the chance of recovery. Rapid discharge from ICU is not necessarily cost-effective. In some instances, an extra day in ICU may decrease the likelihood of repeat ICU admission and facilitate faster discharge from hospital.

At present only half the patients admitted to ICU with multi-organ failure survive beyond 1 month. At 1 year only a quarter are alive, and only half of these are out of hospital. In order to make better use of ICU resources consideration about long-term benefit and quality of life is required.

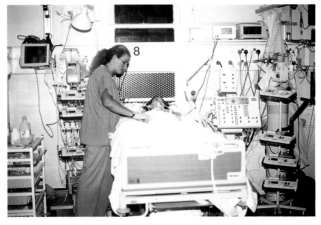

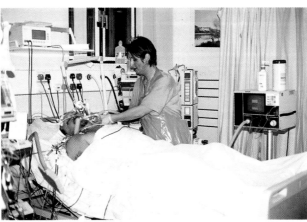

Fig. 1 **Specialist equipment and high staff : patient ratio are some of the distinctive features of an ICU.**

Preoperative optimization

There is increasing data demonstrating the importance of patient optimization prior to proceeding to theatre for major surgery. This is normally undertaken in the ICU, HDU or anaesthetic area. Papers have addressed the role of fluids and vasoactive agents to optimize oxygen delivery and these strategies

Table 1 **Criteria for pre-arrest admission to the ICU.**

Any three of the following:

Central nervous system	Not fully alert and orientated, with oxygen saturation > 90%
Respiratory system	Respiratory rate ≤ 30 or ≤ 10 breaths/minute
Cardiovascular system	Systolic blood pressure ≤ 90 mmHg, and heart rate ≤ 110 or ≤ 55 bpm
Renal system	Urine output < 100 ml over the last 4 hours
OR	
Central nervous system	Not fully alert and orientated, and one of the following: Respiratory rate ≥ 35 breaths/minute Heart rate ≥ 140 bpm

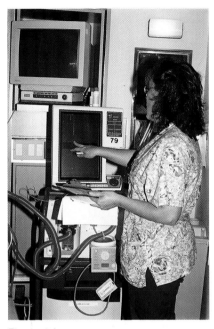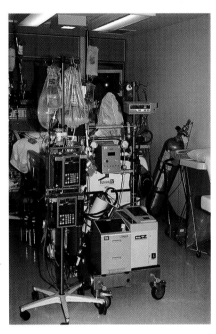

Fig. 3a & b **There have been major advances in artificial ventilation and oxygenation.**
These photographs depict a modern sophisticated mechanical ventilator and a machine that oxygenates blood outside the body, an extra-corporeal membrane oxygenator.

Clinical case 40

Mr D is a 55-year-old man. Consider at what stage the course of his illness could have been predicted, what interventions may have been undertaken and when he should have been admitted to the ICU or HDU to optimize therapy.

Day 1 Mr D presents with constipation and a history of diverticular disease. Clinical findings are of an acute abdomen. He proceeds to laparotomy where he is found to have an acute appendicitis with peritonitis. An appendicetomy is performed and he is transferred to the surgical ward. He has two peripheral lines and a urinary catheter. He is cefuroxime and metronidazole i.v. and analgesia is achieved with opiates and NSAIDs.

Day 2 He is generally unwell, with a distended abdomen (T = 38.5°C, HR = 130 bpm, BP = 100/70, Resp. Rate = 18 breaths/min, urine output 30 ml/hour, blood gases normal: pH 7.39, PCO_2 4.5, PO_2 12, HCO_3 22, saturations 98%). Given more fluids and antibiotics. Creatinine 150 (normal < 120) μmol/l.

Day 3 More unwell with increasing abdominal distension (T = 38.5°C, HR 140, BP 90/60, RR 22, urine output 20 ml/hour, blood gases: pH 7.35, PCO_2 3.5, PO_2 11, HCO_3 16, Base Deficit 8, saturations 96%). Given more fluids and continue antibiotics. Nasogastric tube on free drainage (1 litre/day). Creatinine 190 μmol/l.

Day 4 Very unwell with increasing distension (T = 38.5°C, HR 140, BP 90/40, RR 36, urine output 20 ml/hour, blood gases: pH 7.32, PCO_2 3.0, PO_2 8.0, HCO_3 14, BD 10, saturations 91%). Give oxygen and stop iv fluids. Abdominal X-ray – ileus – continue free drainage. Creatinine 250 μmol/l.

Day 5 Cardiorespiratory arrest, resuscitated and transferred to ICU. Anuric, mean arterial pressure 45.

See comment on page 126.

have been associated with improved outcome and decreased morbidity. Although such facilities are not yet routinely available, the importance of adequate fluid therapy prior to surgery cannot be over-emphasized.

Pre-arrest admission

The concept of 'pre-arrest teams' is becoming more popular. Instead of waiting until a patient becomes haemodynamically unstable and suffers a cardiac arrest, a team could identify and evaluate patients 'at risk' and admit them to ICU if those caring for the patient deem this appropriate (see Table 1). Approximately half of all patients who have a cardiac arrest on the general medical and surgical wards have abnormal vital signs during the 24 hours prior to the arrest. Early identification of these patients and admission to ICU may improve prognosis.

Table 2 **Common reasons for ICU admission**

Head injury
Encephalopathy and seizures
Severe pneumonia
Asthma
Acute respiratory distress syndrome (ARDS)
Pulmonary embolus
Heart failure
Liver failure
Major trauma
Following major surgery
Burns
Sepsis
Poisoning
Drug overdose
Endocrine emergencies
Complications of pregnancy (e.g. eclampsia)

What is intensive care?

- The ICU caters for patients with severe organ dysfunction, who have a reasonable prognosis with optimal treatment.

- Early recognition of patients who may benefit from ICU admission may improve outcome.

- High-risk surgical patients benefit from preoperative treatment in ICU.

- Prognosis is improved when patients are admitted to ICU before cardiac arrest, as opposed to following acute resuscitation.

Organ support

Admission to an intensive care unit (ICU) or high-dependency unit (HDU) allows a higher level of care and monitoring to be employed than can be provided on the general ward. Usually, ICUs provide one-to-one nursing, comprehensive monitoring (including invasive pressures and blood gas analysis) and organ support (mechanical ventilation, extra-corporeal oxygenation, intra-aortic counter pulsation and renal dialysis (see Fig. 1).

Critically ill patients either have severe impairment of one organ system or impairment of more than one system. The management of critically ill patients in ICU is best achieved by a multidisciplinary team.

ICU multidisciplinary team

- Primary referring team, intensivists and intensive care nurses.
- Support services specialists (radiology, microbiology, biochmemistry and haematology).
- Pharamacist, physiotherapist and dietician.
- Medical equipment technicians and receptionist.

Respiratory support

Timing and nature of respiratory intervention is based both on the degree of abnormality of the gas exchange and on the trends in the physiological variables.

Indications for respiratory support include:

- Hypoxia.
- Hypercarbia.
- Failure to protect airway (neurological).
- Local trauma (eg laryngeal trauma, facial fractures, glottic oedema).
- Increased work of breathing (eg metabolic complications, chest wall abnormalities)

Respiratory support may be classified as simple, non-invasive or advanced. Non-invasive mask ventilation and continuous positive airway pressure (CPAP) can normally be provided in the HDU, while advanced ventilatory support requires ICU.

For advanced ventilatory techniques, tracheal intubation is required. This is normally achieved via the oral route in the first instance but progression to a

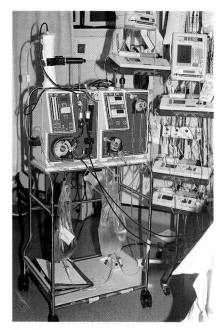

Fig. 1 **A dialysis machine, one means by which organ support can be provided, in this case to the kidneys.**

tracheostomy may be necessary for patients who are likely to require intubation for longer than 7 days. To facilitate both patient comfort and adequate ventilation, sedative and analgesic drugs are normally used, at least in the initial stages of ICU care. The following are frequently used, either alone or in combination, for this purpose: morphine, fentanyl, midazolam, propofol.

There are many techniques to provide ventilatory support and patients may experience several of these during a stay in ICU. Patients may breathe spontaneously via a ventilator, have a mixture of spontaneous and mechanical ventilation or be totally ventilator-dependent. Mechanical ventilation may be delivered in volume- or pressure-determined mode.

For example, in acute respiratory distress syndrome (ARDS) standard management includes intermittent positive pressure ventilation (IPPV) with positive end-expiratory pressure (PEEP), aimed at providing adequate oxygenation ($PaO_2 > 8$ kPa), while avoiding excessive pressure (barotrauma) applied or excessive volume (volutrauma) delivered to the lungs (see Fig. 2). Often in these patients mechanical ventilation is best delivered using small tidal volumes (5 ml/kg) at a higher rate, allowing carbon dioxide to build up to an acceptable level (permissive hypercapnia > 7 kPa).

Cardiovascular support

The methods of cardiovascular support are determined by the cause of the cardiovascular failure. Shock is a well-defined form of extreme cardiovascular failure dealt with in 'Shock' on page 76.

Circulatory instability due to hypovolaemia requires urgent fluid replacement. Haemorrhagic hypovolaemia requires treatment with colloid and packed red cells. If there is

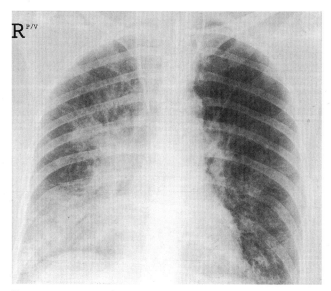

Fig. 2 **Chest X-ray showing bilateral pulmonary infiltrates in a patient with ARDS.** Notice the tracheal tube and central venous catheters.

an accompanying clotting disorder, fresh frozen plasma, cryoprecipitate or platelets may be required.

If cardiac output requires support, consequent to pump failure, inotropic drugs may be needed such as dobutamine or milrinone. In certain circumstances support with an intra-aortic counter-pulsating balloon or a ventricular assist device may be necessary.

Continuous invasive monitoring of arterial blood is mandatory in patients receiving vasoactive agents. These agents should be infused via a central venous catheter, allowing concurrent measurement of central venous pressure. Cardiac output and filling status may be assessed by echocardiography or calculated following insertion of a pulmonary artery flotation catheter.

Renal support

Acid–base status, urea, creatinine and electrolytes must be closely monitored in all patients with developing and established renal dysfunction. The commonest cause of acute renal failure (ARF) in the ICU is acute tubular necrosis, but other causes should always be considered and investigated.

The volume of urine output does not reflect renal function. For example, frusemide and dopamine, following appropriate volume loading, may increase urine output but do not affect the development or the course of an episode of renal failure.

Renal replacement therapy, when required, is achieved by continuous haemofiltration, haemodiafiltration or slow continuous haemodialysis. Intermittent haemodialysis is poorly tolerated in the haemodynamically fragile patient and plays a part only in stable patients with isolated renal failure. There is a trend towards early institution of renal support in patients with sepsis and ARF, rather than waiting for the traditional indicators (acidosis, hyperkalaemia, uraemia or fluid overload).

Support of the central nervous system

The Glasgow Coma Scale (see Appendix) and pupillary response to light should be assessed regularly. Interpretation of these signs, however, must take into account the effect of sedative or other drugs. Neuromuscular blockade will obviously render assessment of motor and verbal response impossible.

In patients at risk of raised intracranial pressure (ICP), invasive monitoring may be instituted to measure ICP and cerebral perfusion pressure (CPP, defined as the difference between mean arterial pressure and ICP). Raised ICP should be treated surgically if possible. Mannitol (50–100 g iv) temporarily reduces ICP. CPP can be maintained using drugs to optimize blood pressure. Psychological aspects of the ICU care are important and are covered on page 112.

Immune function and infections

Patients in the ICU are often immunocompromised and care should be taken to prevent cross-infection between patients and minimize nosocomial infections. Particularly important in this aspect is the adherence to hand washing and equipment cleaning (e.g. stethoscopes) between patients.

Gastrointestinal support and feeding

The patient's nutritional status must be considered, as trauma, surgery and sepsis increase tissue-protein breakdown. In the absence of any gastrointestinal contraindications, patients should be fed enterally. Enteral nutrition provides calories and substrate to the patient and also preserves the integrity and the function of the intestinal mucosa. In intubated patients, enteral feeding may be via a nasogastric tube, but if gastric aspirates are large a post-pyloric tube may be needed.

Parenteral nutrition may be undertaken if enteral nutrition fails but is only rarely required. The incidence of stress ulceration has fallen in recent years with improved resuscitation and early enteral nutrition. Further protection may be obtained with H_2 antagonists, proton pump inhibitors or sucralfate. See also page 47.

Skin and musculoskeletal support

Patients in the ICU require considerable support from nurses, physiotherapists and relatives to maintain movement and prevent development of contractures and skin lesions. Modern beds and improved skin-care and nutrition have decreased the incidence of pressure sores.

Neuromuscular blocking drugs are only rarely indicated in ICU patients. If their use is unavoidable (eg. failure to oxygenate in status asthmaticus, status epilepticus or severe tetanus) it must be ensured that paralysed patients receive adequate sedation to guarantee unconsciousness.

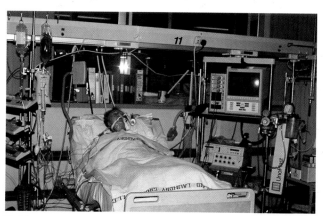

Fig. 3 **An ICU patient surrounded by an array of monitors and devices to provide organ support.**

Organ support

- ICU provides multidisciplinary expertise that is not available elsewhere.
- Temporary organ support allows for recovery from the underlying insult.
- Interventions are available to supplement function of all major organ systems.
- Lungs, kidneys, liver, heart and even brain function may recover markedly.

Monitoring of the ICU patient

Patients in the ICU and HDU environment are frequently unstable, and appropriate monitoring is important to delineate trends in the patient's physiological status. Monitoring per se is not a goal, rather it guides interventions aiming to prevent organ damage and to promote recovery.

Because care in the ICU is primarily directed at sustaining life, delivery of oxygen and other substrates to the tissues is of the utmost importance. Therefore, a large proportion of available monitoring is centred around the circulatory and respiratory systems.

Electrocardiogram (ECG)

Lawrie demonstrated in 1967 that ECG monitoring decreased mortality by 20% in patients with myocardial infarction by facilitating immediate defibrillation for ventricular fibrillation. All patients in ICU/HDU are severely ill or highly dependent on interventions, thus requiring ECG monitoring because of the risk of arrhythmias.

Examples of arrhythmia precipitants:

- Myocardial ischaemia/infarction.
- Cardiotoxic drugs.
- Acute neurological dysfunction (stroke, head injury, encephalitis).
- Metabolic disarray, severe hypoxia, hypercarbia or acidosis.
- Electrolyte disturbances, especially plasma potassium.
- Cardiovascular instability (trauma, postoperative, sepsis).
- Following coronary angioplasty.
- Renal failure or fluid balance problems.

Pulse oximetry

Measurement is normally taken using a finger or toe probe but there are also probes for use on the earlobe, nose and mouth. The principles of the measurement are described in 'Oximetry and capnography' on page 54. Pulse oximetry only monitors oxygenation of arterial blood and provides no measure of ventilation or carbon dioxide concentration.

Arterial blood gas analysis

A modern blood gas analysis utilizes electrochemical techniques to measure pH, PCO_2 and PO_2. All modern blood gas machines are provided with a computer that contains a set of buffer curves for human blood and calculates bicarbonate and base deficit/excess based on the haemoglobin content of blood.

The technique of blood gas analysis requires anaerobic sampling of blood into a heparinized 2 ml syringe. Samples may be taken from an indwelling arterial catheter or by means of a direct 'stab' of a peripheral artery, usually the femoral or the radial arteries (page 58). Sampling of blood from an indwelling arterial catheter through a long plastic tube requires the disposal of the 'dead space' of saline normally filling the tube into another (10 ml) syringe (Fig. 3).

Pressure measurements

Arterial blood pressure monitoring may be undertaken intermittently using a sphygmomanometer. In ICU/HDU

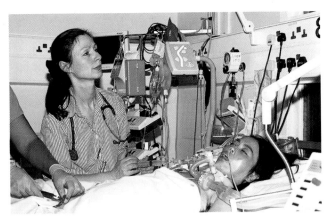

Fig. 1 **ICU doctor measuring cardiac output.**

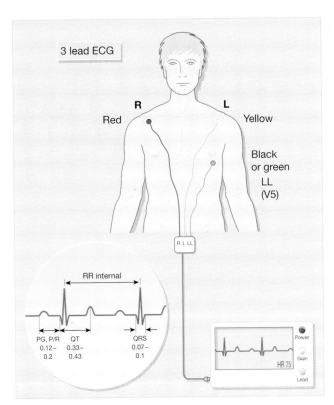

Fig. 2 **Three-lead ECG.** Correct positioning of electrodes.

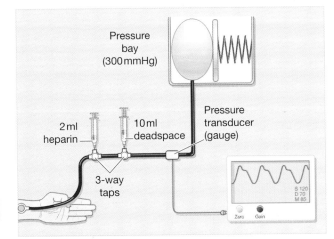

Fig. 3 **Indwelling arterial catheter.**

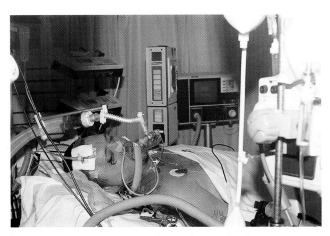

Fig. 4 **An intracranial bolt can be used to monitor intracranial pressure.**

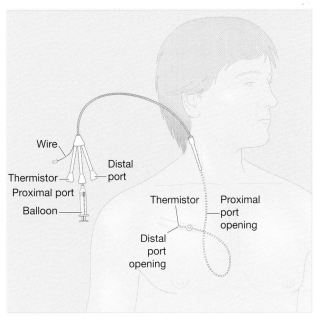

Fig. 5 **Continuous invasive pressure monitoring system.**

continuous invasive pressure monitoring is more useful. The same system may be used for monitoring arterial, central venous (CVP), pulmonary artery (PAP), or intracranial (ICP) pressures (Fig. 4). It provides a trace and dynamic measurements of pressures.

The components required are a transducer, a fluid-filled catheter, a flush device and an appropriate monitoring system. It is important to understand the physical properties and to be capable of zeroing and calibrating the system. Invasive arterial pressure monitoring is indicated in haemodynamically unstable patients. Arterial cannulation also provides a port for regular sampling of blood for gas analysis. There is a risk of exsanguination should the line be left open.

Central venous cannulation provides a route for the safe and speedy delivery of drugs and fluids and measurement of CVP provides a guide to intravascular volume.

Pulmonary artery catheterization with a special 'floating' catheter allows measurement of PAP, pulmonary capillary wedge pressure (PCWP, an estimate of left atrial pressure), and cardiac output (Fig. 5). Some catheters are provided with a fibre-optic channel allowing measurement of mixed venous saturation.

Temperature

Core temperature may be measured from a pulmonary artery catheter or from a tympanic, oesophageal, nasopharyngeal, rectal or bladder probe. 'Peripheral' temperature is usually measured over the toe or the dorsal aspect of the foot and is used as an indication of peripheral perfusion rather than of heat homeostasis (see also page 34).

Capnography

Capnography provides breath-by-breath analysis of carbon dioxide in expired gas (see Oximetry and capnography, pages 54–55). Since end-tidal and arterial CO_2 are usually very close, capnography is useful in ventilated patients without frequent recourse to blood gas analysis.

Neurological

Intracranial pressure (ICP) monitoring is useful following head injury to guide the management of raised ICP and for optimization of cerebral perfusion pressure (see Fig. 4). The probe may be placed in the extradural, subdural, parenchymal

or ventricular compartments. The adequacy of cerebral perfusion may also be judged from measurement of jugular bulb venous blood oxygen saturations. The insertion of micro dialysis probes or special catheters with a PO_2 sensitive tip or miniaturized thermocouples into the substance of the brain to assess tissue oxygenation and temperature are new and evolving techniques not yet widely used.

Clinical case 41

A 55-year-old presented with a history of haematemesis. He received 2L of Ringer's lactate solution through two peripheral catheters, but remained cold and shut-down. Observations revealed: pulse 140, sinus rhythm, blood pressure 90/50 lying, 70/40 sitting. Pulse oximetry applied to the finger showed an intermittent trace with saturations of 91% despite oxygen by facemask. A central venous catheter was inserted with difficulty under local anaesthetic to guide volume replacement. The CVP was 4 mmHg. It was decided to perform a gastric endoscopy. Pulse oximetry indicated a saturation of 89–90% but since the trace was of poor quality, it was thought not to represent the patients' true status. ECG monitoring was instituted and 5 mg of midazolam was given to alleviate agitation. Saturation readings decreased to 85%. The patient struggled as the endoscopy proceeded. He vomited and became cyanosed. The endoscopy was abandoned and a tracheal tube was inserted to protect the airway and provide oxygen. Comment on this sequence of events.
See comment on page 126–127.

Monitoring the ICU patient

- The blind institution of monitoring does not improve survival and may result in morbidity.
- Monitoring is intended to help with the provision of organ support and to allow rapid recognition of changes in the patient's condition.
- Monitoring is useful when staff are able to interpret and act upon the information provided.
- Monitoring does not replace clinical acumen and judgement.
- It is important to know the limitations, applications and appropriateness of various monitors.

Brain death and organ donation

Brain death

Brain death signifies the total and irreversible loss of all brain function, including that of the brain stem. The brain stem function is the essential component of the brain required to sustain life. Before the advent of intensive care units with the facility for artificial ventilation, cessation of cardiac activity accompanied brain stem death. Patients would have stopped breathing immediately following a primary brain injury, and asystole would have occurred within minutes.

Patients with severe brain damage who are deeply unconscious may still retain the capacity to breathe. These patients are in a persistent vegetative state with some brain stem function, and as such are not dead. The diagnosis of death carries important medicolegal, ethical, cultural and philosophical considerations. In many Western cultures loss of the potential to regain consciousness or breathe again are accepted as evidence of death. Therefore brain stem death equates to death. This is a difficult concept to appreciate as it occurs before circulatory arrest, but it is notable that no patient fulfilling the diagnostic criteria for brain stem death has ever regained consciousness. Simply stated, death is a process and not an event. Once the process has progressed beyond death of the brain stem, there is no return.

Brain stem functions

- Respiratory drive.
- Blood pressure maintenance.
- Arousal centre – ability to be conscious.
- All motor output.
- Most sensory input.
- Autonomic efferents pass through.
- Cranial nerve reflexes.

Diagnosis

The diagnosis of brain stem death is made clinically. It is essential that the condition leading to coma is identified. Likely causes include severe head injury, intracranial haemorrhage, prolonged cardiac arrest, and brain tumour. Once this primary diagnosis has been made, the necessary preconditions and exclusion criteria can be applied.

The computerized tomography (CT) scans in Figure 1 show an example of an injury to the brain resulting in irreversible structural damage. The scan of the head with contrast shows a large intracranial bleed (Fig. 1a) and secondary hydrocephalus (Fig. 1b).

Preconditions to diagnosing death are:

- A condition leading to irreversible structural brain damage is identified.
- The patient is unconscious and artificially ventilated.

Exclusion criteria include reversible changes to brain stem function, which may be caused by a number of drugs and metabolic disturbances. Before making the diagnosis of brain stem death, doctors need to be satisfied that there is no reversible component to the coma. Therefore the following should be excluded before testing for brain stem death:

- Drug intoxication.
- Sedation.
- Neuromuscular blockade.
- Hypothermia (< 35°C).
- Biochemical derangement
- Recent convulsions.

Time of testing

Once any doubt that the condition is irremediable has been ruled out, testing can begin. This means that time to testing will vary as time taken to fulfil preconditions and exclusion criteria varies. For example, deterioration of a neurosurgical patient in hospital with evidence of a second intracranial haemorrhage, may be tested within hours. Cerebral hypoxia secondary to cardiac arrest may require 24 hours to ensure the irreversible nature of brain damage. Suspected drug

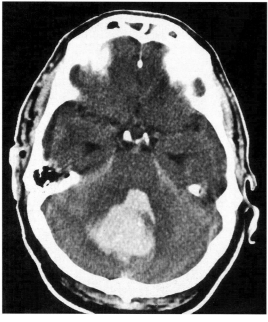

(a)

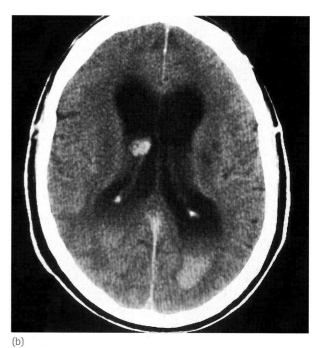

(b)

Fig. 1 **(a) CT scan showing intracranial haemorrhage and (b) secondary hydrocephalus.**

intoxication may take longer, depending on the half-life of the drugs in question. Clinical judgement needs to be applied to each individual case.

Testing

Two doctors of sufficient experience, one a consultant, the other at least 5 years post-registration, should carry out the tests. Two sets of tests should be carried out. There is no fixed interval between the tests, and clinical judgement needs to be employed.

The equipment in Figure 2 is required for brain stem death verification.

Tests

Once each doctor is satisfied that preconditions and exclusion criteria have been met, testing of brain stem reflexes may begin. The pupils should remain unreactive on shining a bright light directly into each eye. If atropine has been given (even several hours previously) this test is invalid. Pre-existing pupil abnormalities should be ruled out. Corneal reflexes should be absent after corneal stimulation with a swab.

Caloric testing confirms absence of vestibulo-ocular reflexes. First the tympanic membrane must be visualized on inspection of the auditory canal. This may require removal of any wax obscuring the view. After instillation of ice-cold water (20 ml) directly towards each tympanic membrane, there should be no eye movements. Absence of motor function in the cranial nerve distribution should be confirmed. There should be no facial movement in response to a painful stimulus. Pharyngeal and tracheal stimulation should fail to elicit any gag or cough reflex.

Apnoea testing confirms the diagnosis of brain stem death. The patient should be ventilated with 100% oxygen for 10 minutes before carrying out this test, so as to avoid hypoxia (which may itself affect brain function). The $PaCO_2$ prior to disconnection should be around 5.3 kPa (40 mmHg). After discontinuation of artificial ventilation, oxygen should be insufflated down the tracheal tube via a catheter at 6 l/minute. The absence of any respiratory movement during the period of apnoea substantiates the diagnosis. $PaCO_2$ at the end of the period of close observation must be shown to have reached a level which should be sufficient to drive respiration (> 6.5 kPa (50 mmHg) in the UK).

Time of death is the time at which the first set of brain stem death tests is completed. After completion of the second set of tests the decision to cease artificial ventilation is made.

Brain stem death

- NO pupil response to light.
- NO corneal reflex.
- NO vestibulo-ocular reflex.
- NO cranial nerve motor function.
- NO gag reflex.
- NO cough reflex.
- NO breathing efforts.

Organ donation

A patient who has been declared brain stem-dead is a potential organ donor. The patient's next of kin must give consent to retrieval of suitable organs. Good communication among medical staff, relatives, transplant coordinators and nursing staff is of the utmost importance during this difficult period, and time must be allowed for relatives to come to terms with their recent loss.

The transplant team requires a full medical history, details of medication given and results of biochemical, haematological, bacteriological and viral investigations, as well as a recent chest X-ray and electrocardiogram.

Care of the potential organ donor continues in the intensive care unit.

Major cardiovascular instability may occur in the brain stem-dead patient, and management should be directed towards maintaining organ perfusion and oxygenation. Fluid therapy, inotropic support, temperature control and antibiotic prophylaxis may be required.

The operation for retrieval of organs sometimes causes a haemodynamic response similar to that seen in inadequately anaesthetized patients. Muscle-relaxant drugs are occasionally given during retrieval to abolish movement caused by spinal reflexes. Controversy surrounds the question of whether anaesthetic drugs should be administered to organ donors. Haemodynamic responses and spinal reflexes do not imply consciousness. Indeed if the remotest possibility of consciousness was contemplated, organ donation would be highly inappropriate. The most convincing argument for providing anaesthetic drugs and muscle relaxants is that the abolition of these responses may decrease the emotional discomfort of those who are present while the organs are removed.

Clinical case 42

A 60-year-old man presented with decreased conscious level following a severe headache. His Glasgow Coma score was 7 on admission. He was given sedative drugs and muscle relaxants prior to tracheal intubation and ventilation. CT scan revealed an extensive intracranial haemorrhage. His condition deteriorated, blood pressure increased and heart rate decreased. He was unresponsive and his pupils were noted to be fixed and dilated. What should be done?
See comment on page 127.

Brain death and organ donation

- Death is a process, not an event.
- Always make a primary diagnosis of brain injury.
- Apply preconditions and exclusion criteria.
- No brain stem-dead patient has ever recovered.
- Any brain stem-dead patient is a candidate for organ donation.

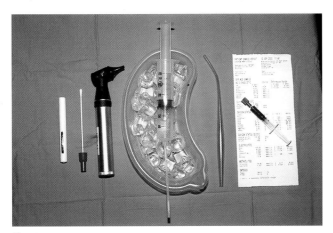

Fig. 2 **Equipment required for brain stem testing.**

Psychological aspects of ICU

The intensive care unit appears to be a comfortable work environment for its regular staff. In reality, however, it is in many aspects a profoundly alien environment not only to patients and relatives, but also to medical and paramedical staff who do not routinely work on intensive care units.

In all medical practice holistic care of the patient is paramount. In the critical care arena the responsibility is even greater. The multidisciplinary team must provide excellence of care in all its different aspects, and truly act as the patient's advocate. In contrast to normal clinical situations, the patient is frequently unable to communicate and is thus prohibited from participation in decisions regarding their care. All members of the healthcare team have responsibility for the safe and appropriate care of each vulnerable patient on the ICU. Optimal care is achieved when team members communicate effectively. This communication must be with the patient, their relatives and friends, the referring and reviewing clinical teams and all members of the multidisciplinary team.

Environment

The first and often most striking finding on visiting and ICU/HDU area is that immediate access is denied. Although this is instituted for a variety of appropriate reasons, it may be frustrating to relatives and visiting medical teams alike. The reasons should be explained and a good intercom system may prevent some frustration. Comfortable waiting areas for relatives should be provided in addition to quiet secluded rooms that may be used to discuss patients' progress.

Upon entering the ICU one is confronted by a barrage of stimuli (see Fig. 1). There is a cacophony of alarms and bleeps, and a spectacle of bright flashing lights and traces from the array of monitoring systems. Doctors, nurses, physiotherapists, pharmacists, technicians and students appear to mill around. An assortment of equipment may render difficult approach to the bedside of the profoundly ill patient.

All this is very distressing to relatives and friends who last saw their loved one sitting on a ward or indeed as healthy individuals at home. The biggest shock is usually seeing the patient unconscious and connected to a mechanical ventilator, an image associated by many with inevitable death. It is important to talk to visitors and explain to them what the equipment is for and encourage them to sit with their relative, hold their hands and talk to them. The intensive care nurse has an invaluable role in facilitating this.

Friends and family

Relatives and visitors should be made to feel comfortable when visiting and be provided with regular updates about the patient's progress by the nursing and medical staff. Nonetheless, it is also important to recognize the patient's right to confidentiality when deciding upon the amount and appropriateness of information given.

Relatives and friends suffer profound stress from having loved ones in critical care areas. The need to face mortality, the inability to predict progress, repeated setbacks, travelling to and from hospital and the financial burden all take their toll on individuals and families.

It is sad but inevitable that many patients die in the ICU. As such an inherent part of ICU care is to provide appropriate care for dying patients and to help the family with bereavement. This is difficult in the alienating ICU environment, and most staff are not adequately trained for these roles.

The patient

The patient, who is the central player in all of this activity, is initially nearly always sedated to facilitate optimal management, in particular mechanical ventilation of the lungs. The sedation is decreased to allow weaning off ventilation support. This process may be traumatic as patients become aware of their circumstances and the discomfort may be compounded by drug withdrawal syndromes.

The patient has to cope with bright lights, loud noises, sleep deprivation and insertion of lines and tubes (see Fig. 2). Loss of normal circadian rhythm frequently occurs. In addition many have limited mobility, both because they are restricted by

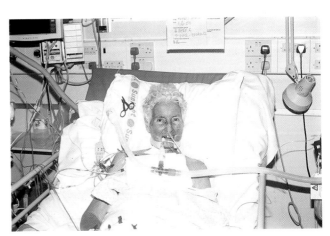

Fig. 1 **Upon entering the ICU one is confronted by a barrage of stimuli: a cacophony of alarms and bleeps, and a spectacle of bright flashing lights and traces of monitoring systems.**

Fig. 2 **A patient who is awake but still has a tracheal tube in place. She is alert, comfortable and able to communicate.**

monitors and intravenous lines and also related to muscle weakness that many patients experience.

Communication with relatives is, as has been mentioned, of great importance, but above and beyond this, it is essential to talk to the patient. Auditory awareness is the last sense to be depressed by sedative drugs. As such, patients may be aware of conversations taking place around the bedside making polite and appropriate discussions mandatory. In addition it is common courtesy when approaching any patient, whether sedated or awake, to introduce oneself and explain what you are going to do especially with regard to physical examination.

A recent study looked at 227 patients who had been discharged from a general ICU. At 3 months 80% of the patients interviewed were satisfied with their quality of life, the prevalence of psychological distress was low; 12% had heightened anxiety and nearly 10% were depressed. There were high levels of poor concentration, fatigue and sleep disturbance. These symptoms improved over the next 9 months. None of this should surprise us. In fact, when healthy volunteers are placed in an ICU environment for 4 days they develop feelings of depression, fatigue and confusion. Patients who are admitted to the ICU are even more likely to experience such feelings related to their dependency and physical frailty.

The term ICU psychosis has been used to describe a cluster of psychiatric symptoms that are unique to the ICU environment. It is postulated that many aspects of the ICU environment may contribute, such as sensory overload, pain, presence of tubes and lines, sleep deprivation, time disorientation and inability to communicate and/or understand the sequence of events that have taken place. In addition, organic stresses may contribute to a confused state, such as ongoing systemic sepsis and withdrawal of sedative drugs. Patients may continue to have dreams, nightmares and post-traumatic stress responses following ICU discharge. Ward staff should be aware of this and arrange appropriate support, including psychiatric referral.

Staff

It is important to communicate regularly with the referring medical teams and also the patient's general practitioner (see Fig. 3). The medical team should feel involved in the care and management of the patient and be aware of progress and plans to facilitate transfer back to the ward at a later date. Discussions with the family doctor help provide community support for family members both during and following the ICU period. All visiting teams to the ICU should be made to feel welcome and relevant to the patients care.

Although ICU and HDU are characteristically referred to as areas of high stress with the potential for 'burnout', there is data to show that stress is not higher than in a normal ward area. There are several strategies that may be undertaken to limit stress and 'burnout'. The ICU/HDU should be made as relaxed and comfortable as possible, preferably with lots of natural light. The feeling of being part of a worthwhile, productive team must be ensured. This is facilitated by open, effective lines of communication within the multidisciplinary team (Fig. 4). Every member of the team is important and their view should be valued, be they a junior staff nurse, consultant, physiotherapist or receptionist. The whole cannot work if the parts are not in harmony. Some units find that regular debriefing and counselling sessions for staff are beneficial.

Clinical follow-up

Increasingly, ICU facilities are arranging follow-up of patients following discharge from ICU. This provides information not only on long-term health problems but also on how the ICU service may be improved for patients and their relatives and friends.

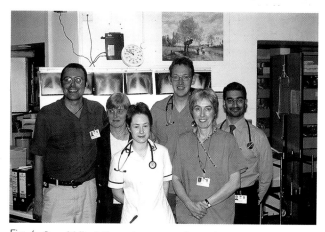

Fig. 4 **A multidisciplinary team on an intensive care unit.**

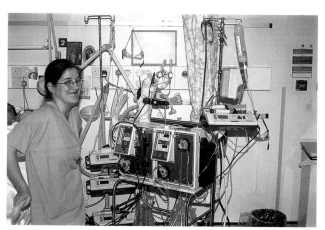

Fig. 3 **The nurse has the most intense contact with the ICU patient, and is frequently best placed to communicate information to other health workers, friends and family.**

> ### Psychological aspects of ICU
>
> - The ICU is an alienating environment for patients, visitors and many staff members.
> - Communication among staff members, with patients and with their relatives is of paramount importance.
> - All members of the multidisciplinary team contribute to patient care and the smooth running of a unit.
> - ICU patients frequently suffer from sleep disorders and depression.
> - The psychological consequences of an ICU admission may only become apparent on the ward following discharge.

Emergency airway management

When a person has impaired breathing there is a window of opportunity, during which appropriate intervention may avert disaster and result in a favourable outcome. Doctors in training are often called upon to intervene in such a crisis on the wards. A simple approach to assisting with ventilation and facilitating airflow to the lungs may be life-saving (see Fig. 1). Emergency airway management may be required in the following instances:

- Unconscious patients who cannot maintain airway patency or protect their lungs from aspiration of gastric contents, for example, immediately following surgery under general anaesthesia.
- Following an overdose with drugs that depress ventilation, such as opiates and sedatives, both of which are frequently administered during endoscopic procedures.
- Patients who have breathing difficulties as may occur with asthma, chronic lung disease, pneumonia and muscle weakness.
- Patients who have had a cardiac arrest.

Call for help early

Oxygenation is the main priority. Hospital doctors should have a simple plan of action to provide oxygen should they encounter a patient with a compromised airway. It is vital to appreciate when advanced airway management is required, for which the on-call anaesthetist should be called immediately, before the patient has a cardiac arrest.

A stepwise plan
- Relieve airway obstruction: suction food and vomit and attempt to facilitate airflow (chin lift, jaw thrust).

- Assist ventilation:
  - Mask to mouth.
  - Self-inflating bag and mask.
- Provide supplementary oxygen.
- Promote airway patency.

The following methods of promoting airway patency are listed according to training required:

- Oropharyngeal airway
- Nasopharyngeal airway
- Laryngeal mask airway (LMA)

The definitive conduit for facilitating ventilation and protecting against aspiration of gastric contents is a cuffed tracheal (or tracheostomy) tube. Insertion requires an advanced level of training and regular practice, and should not be attempted by unskilled doctors in an emergency situation.

Provision of oxygen

Whenever possible all forms of emergency assisted ventilation should be with the highest attainable concentration of inspired oxygen.

Optimal use of bag and mask

Except for those with advanced training (e.g. anaesthetists) optimal use of a bag and mask (Fig. 2) requires two people. One person maintains a patent airway by applying a chin lift while ensuring an airtight seal between the mask and the patient's face (Fig. 3). An oropharyngeal airway may prevent the tongue from obstructing airflow. The second person inflates the lungs by compression of the bag at a rate of 12 breaths per minute or, if CPR is in progress, at a rate of one bag compression to every five

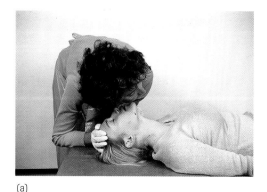

(a)

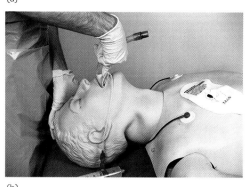

(b)

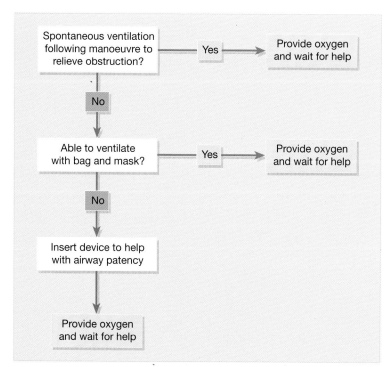

Fig. 1 **An approach to the patient with breathing difficulties.**

chest compressions. It is not necessary to empty the bag with each squeeze; visible chest expansion is a suitable end point. Overzealous squeezing of the bag results in gastric distension with the subsequent risk of regurgitation and aspiration of stomach contents.

The laryngeal mask airway

The laryngeal mask airway (LMA) is used for the majority of anaesthetics in the UK. Following insertion, the soft silicon bowl of the LMA rests beyond the tongue in the larynx, allowing unobstructed breathing and assisted ventilation. The LMA has enjoyed widespread success for the following reasons: it is inserted without the need for a laryngoscope. Competent LMA insertion is possible following brief training. The majority of LMA insertions are successful. The LMA is well tolerated by a lightly sedated or semiconscious patient; it has been widely accepted as a first-line airway device for use in resuscitation.

The major disadvantage of the LMA is that it does not protect the lungs from soiling with gastric contents. Furthermore, it is not designed as a conduit for subsequent insertion of a tracheal tube. Modifications of the LMA that might improve these shortcomings are presently undergoing clinical trials. See Fig. 1b for LMA insertion technique.

Assisting with intubation

When the anaesthetist has to insert a tracheal tube (Fig. 4) under pressure in an emergency, a colleague familiar with the equipment and able to provide help in the following ways is invaluable: Assist with ventilation and the provision of oxygen; ensure that essential equipment is functional and available; lubricate the tube and cuff with water-soluble jelly. Present a working laryngoscope to the anaesthetist's left hand and the tracheal tube to the right hand. Apply cricoid pressure when requested (see Fig. 4). Inflate the cuff with 5 ml of air after insertion of the tracheal tube. Connect the tube to bag with an oxygen supply.

Confirming position of the tracheal tube

The following suggest that a tracheal tube is likely to be in the trachea:

- Auscultation over the lung fields reveals breath sounds at the lung apices and in the axillae, but not over the stomach.
- Carbon dioxide is detected during exhalation.

There remains the possibility that the tracheal tube has been advanced too far and its tip lies in one of the main bronchi (common) or it has been left above the vocal cords (uncommon). If in doubt, remove the tube and adopt an alternative plan to provide oxygenation until a more experienced doctor arrives.

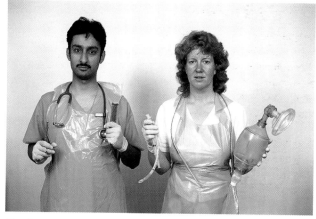

Fig. 4 **Photograph showing the equipment necessary for intubation.** One person is holding the metal items (laryngoscope, stethoscope and Magill's forceps), and the other has the plastic items (tracheal tube with syringe, suction catheter and self-inflating bag).

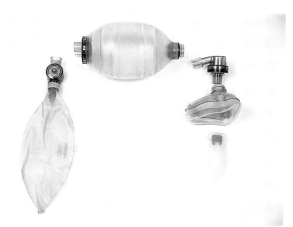

Fig. 2 **Components of a self-inflating bag and mask.**

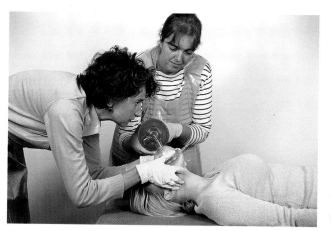

Fig. 3 **Technique for optimal use of a bag and mask.**

Clinical case 43

A patient has become unconscious and stopped breathing on the surgical ward after returning from the operating theatre. Carotid pulses are clearly present. Initially, ventilation was successful with a bag and mask. SHOs has been trying unsuccessfully for 1 minute to insert a tracheal tube. The patient is developing a blue tinge and the heart rate is decreasing. What should be done?
See comment on page 127.

Emergency airway management

- All doctors must have a simple plan for emergency airway management.
- The priority is oxygenation of the lungs, not intubation of the trachea.
- The LMA should be used when the skill to intubate the trachea is not available.
- The tracheal tube protects the lungs from soiling.

Resuscitation

Cardiopulmonary arrest is the sudden loss of effective cardiac and pulmonary function, leading rapidly to unconsciousness and death if not reversed. Neurological damage can occur within minutes if effective circulation and ventilation are not restored.

The majority of cardiac arrests are due to sudden ventricular fibrillation (VF). A direct current (DC) shock (defibrillation) promptly delivered to the chest wall is the treatment of choice. The success of a defibrillation decreases 5–10% for every minute from the onset of VF. When defibrillation is promptly available, the survival figures at 28 days after a cardiac arrest are 12% for out-of-hospital arrests and 39% for in-hospital arrests. Doctors and other hospital workers should be trained in effective resuscitation.

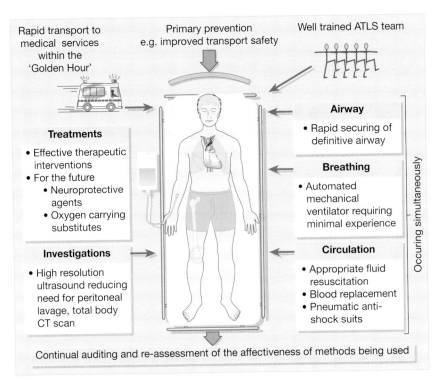

Fig. 1 **Trauma resuscitation into the 21st century.**

CPR

CPR stands for cardiopulmonary resuscitation and encompasses chest compressions and ventilation of the lungs, the combination of which ensures that some blood flows through vital organs, in particular the brain, to prevent irreversible ischaemic injury (see Fig. 1).

Chest compressions

The effect of chest compressions is to propel blood through some of the vital organs. The mechanism by which this is achieved is not fully understood but squeezing of the heart and rapidly increasing and decreasing intra-thoracic pressure are important factors.

Even when performed optimally, only 10–15% of normal cardiac output is achieved. When a tracheal tube is in place, the end tidal carbon dioxide concentration ($ETCO_2$) is a guide to effectiveness of chest compressions and indicates prognosis. An $ETCO_2$ less than 2 KPa (15 mmHg) reflects a low cardiac output and is associated with a poor outcome. After one minute of chest compression fatigue begins to limit its effectiveness.

Oxygenation

A patent airway is essential to maintain oxygenation (see page 114). It is important to reiterate that the aim is oxygenation and not tracheal intubation, as is sometimes suggested, and that the most readily available and familiar airway adjunct should be used.

Defibrillation

Defibrillation aims to restore sinus rhythm when cardiac electrical activity is chaotic and disorganized, a condition termed ventricular fibrillation. This is achieved by the provision of a short pulse of unidirectional electrical current arising from the discharge of a capacitor, essentially using technology identical to a camera flash.

Team Leader Confirms the cardiac arrest using ABC, coordinates personnel, and decides whether resuscitation should continue

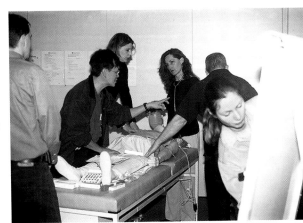

Audit During the arrest a senior person audits events and drugs administered, and reports to and assists the team leader.

Fig. 2 **Teamwork during cardiopulmonary resuscitation.**

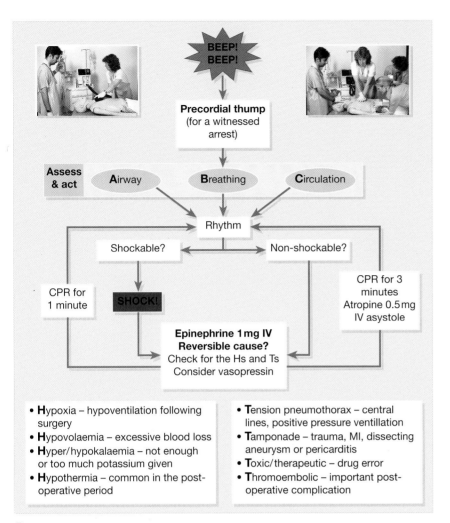

Fig. 3 **Approach to cardiac arrest.**

- **H**ypoxia – hypoventilation following surgery
- **H**ypovolaemia – excessive blood loss
- **H**yper/hypokalaemia – not enough or too much potassium given
- **H**ypothermia – common in the post-operative period

- **T**ension pneumothorax – central lines, positive pressure ventillation
- **T**amponade – trauma, MI, dissecting aneurysm or pericarditis
- **T**oxic/therapeutic – drug error
- **T**hromoembolic – important post-operative complication

Such a pulse resets and synchronizes the refractory periods of the majority of the myocardial cells.

Defibrillators include an electrocardiograph, able to record the ECG from the same paddles that deliver the shock. Most machines rely on the operator's ability to recognize VF and to respond appropriately. Recently, advisory defibrillators have become available with an inclusive computer provided with well-tested software capable of diagnosing the type of arrhythmia and able to deliver defibrillation when indicated.

Successful and appropriate resuscitation

There should be well-trained teams (Fig. 2) and modern working resuscitation equipment throughout the hospital. Patients who are at risk may frequently be identified and monitored in a high-dependency area. Resuscitation may well be inappropriate, especially when prognosis is poor. In such cases, palliative care and counselling are appropriate, and the words 'not for resuscitation' should be written clearly in the notes, with the knowledge of patients and their families.

When a patient sustains a cardiac arrest with ventricular fibrillation within the hospital, defibrillation within minutes is imperative (see Fig. 3). During the provision of CPR, reversible causes of an arrest must be rapidly excluded or treated. If patients do not respond rapidly to resuscitative measures, prognosis is usually poor.

Following successful resuscitation, admission to an intensive care unit is indicated to forestall repeat cardiac arrest and to treat possible complications. Team leaders, in consultation with their colleagues, should have the confidence to make bold decisions. In particular the choice to abandon resuscitation is difficult, but important. Prolonged futile resuscitative efforts are costly and demoralizing.

Clinical case 44

A 67-year-old man has undergone coronary artery bypass surgery. Twelve hours following surgery, he is in the high-dependency unit. There have been numerous ventricluar ectopic beats on the ECG monitor. Having been awake and communicative, he suddenly loses consciousness and the ECG monitor shows ventricular fibrillation. One of the doctors present suggests a precordial thump and immediate CPR. What should be done?
See comment on page 127.

Resuscitation

- The most effective treatment is early defibrillation.
- Exclude the eight reversible causes (the Hs and Ts).
- Coordinated teamwork is crucial.
- Training, practice and familiarity with equipment are key to success.

Drugs and treatment

Many interventions that have been employed during resuscitation have not been evidence-based. In fact, several drugs which were previously administered routinely, may actually worsen outcome. Examples include dextrose, calcium, bicarbonate and lidocaine (lignocaine). In the context of a cardiac arrest, dextrose and calcium may exacerbate ischaemic neurological injury, bicarbonate aggravates intracellular acidosis and lidocaine decreases the likelihood of successful defibrillation. The fact that the medical establishment has been unquestioning about embracing unvalidated interventions in the past is a cautionary note for our current management. Teachers should beware of formulaic teaching and should encourage critical thinking.

Sensible interventions

Besides early defibrillation, there are few interventions associated with improved outcome. All agree that support of circulation and ventilation is indicated, but there is no consensus about the best way to achieve this. Appropriate drug treatment is also subject to intense debate. Even the role of epinephrine (adrenaline), the mainstay of drug therapy, is currently under review. Epinephrine is administered to produce peripheral vasoconstriction, thereby diverting blood to vital organs, in particular the brain (see Fig. 1).

There are other drugs which are powerful vasoconstrictors, (including norepinephrine [noradrenaline, vasopressin and phenylephrine) which may not cause tachycardia when sinus rhythm is restored. There are specific circumstances when particular drugs are indicated. Dextrose, calcium and bicarbonate are all appropriate for the treatment of hyperkalaemia-induced cardiac arrest. Similarly, lidocaine may not treat ventricular fibrillation, but remains useful for the treatment of ventricular arrhythmias and in preventing ventricular fibrillation.

Other useful drugs in a cardiac arrest are specific antidotes. Atropine, for example, is indicated to treat organophosphate poisoning. Information about antidotes may be obtained from a poisons centre.

Defibrillator – tips for use

- Check the defibrillator before a crisis occurs and ensure that it is working and that you understand how to use it (Fig. 2).
- Examine the patient and confirm cardiac arrest.
- Confirm that the ECG leads are applied to the patient's chest.
- Check the ECG monitor. Usually lead 2 is chosen.
- Apply gel pads between the defibrillator paddles and the chest to prevent burns.
- Ensure that the oxygen supply is removed from the bed before delivering a shock (to prevent combustion) (see Fig. 3).
- Charge the paddles only when they are on the patient (Fig. 4).
- Wait for the charge to build before shocking.
- Press both shock buttons simultaneously.
- Do not move charged paddles.
  - If the rhythm is not pulseless ventricular tachycardia or ventricular fibrillation, synchronize the shock with the R wave (by pressing the synch button).
  - Recheck rhythm after each shock.

Controversies in resuscitation

With our ever-increasing ability to extend life beyond its natural limits, much has been said and written in recent years on the subject of resuscitation. Below are some of the controversial areas.

Whom to resuscitate?

Staunch advocates of resuscitation argue that all should receive the benefit of initial resuscitation. Questions may be asked later about the appropriateness of the attempt. Furthermore, each arrest provides excellent training in practical procedures and teamwork.

The converse view is that such an approach may increase the suffering of the patient, squanders valuable resources, and for those with known terminal

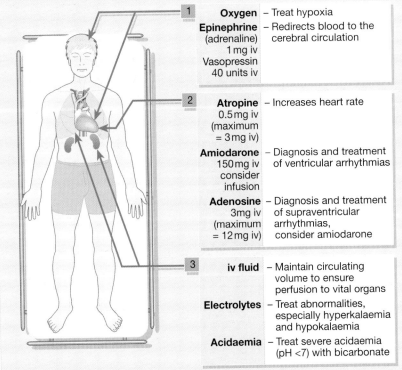

Fig. 1 **Drugs commonly used in resuscitation.** What are we trying to achieve? The three main aimas are 1) perfuse and oxygenate vital organs 2) correct myocardial dysfunction 3) modify biochemical and electrolyte disturbance.

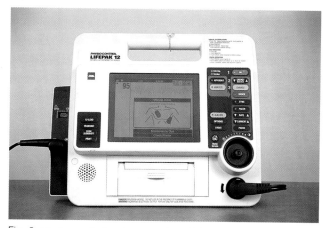

Fig. 2 **Photograph showing a modern defibrillator.**

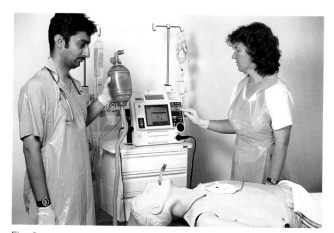

Fig. 3 **Safe use of an advisory defibrillator – note that oxygen is removed.**

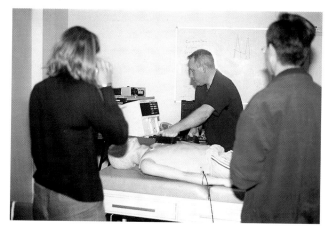

Fig. 4 **Charge the paddles only when they are on the patient, don't move charged paddles.**

illness, regardless of whether the issue has been raised prior to the arrest, resuscitation should not be an option. Additionally, inappropriate resuscitation mandates inappropriate ICU admission and further wastage of resources.

Who should decide about resuscitation?

Some feel that it is doctors' prerogative to decide based on their assessment of prognosis. Others believe this decision should be made only after consultation with the patients and their relatives. Indeed, there are hardliners who maintain that resuscitation should be instituted despite patients' wishes and prognosis.

Should relatives be present during resuscitation?

While for some this may be beneficial to the mourning process, for others it is likely to be highly traumatic and may even jeopardize the likelihood of successful outcome if a distraught relative distracts the team.

'ABC' or 'CAB'?

There is evidence to suggest that the first intervention should be maintenance of circulation (C) rather than airway management (A) and ventilation (B). Chest compression alone with a patent air passage achieves some ventilation. The counter to this is that the 'ABC' approach is easy to remember for the lay person and has been taught in numerous courses.

Are resources appropriately allocated?

In some institutions more that 50% of the postgraduate education budget is spent on resuscitation training. Such training does, however, provide education on broader principles such as pharmacology and teamwork.

Nonetheless, money might be better spent elsewhere, for example funding critical care teams to manage those patients who are seriously ill and at risk of cardiac arrest. There is also the view that spending should be directed towards non-medical staff, for example those who work in the emergency services and in public buildings.

Have there been useful advances?

Proponents of advisory defibrillators claim they are helping save lives in the community. The same is argued about active chest compression decompression devices, which have the appearance of drain plungers. Sceptics remark that there has been minimal improvement in survival despite such technological 'advances', which constitute even further unnecessary expenditure.

Clinical case 45

A 35-year-old single mother was diagnosed with carcinoma of the breast. She underwent mastectomy and axillary-node clearance. Subsequent tests showed liver and bone metastasis, which have responded poorly to therapy. In the past 2 weeks she has become increasingly confused and was admitted to hospital. CT scan of the head is suggestive brain metastases. The patient is unfit presently to give consent on the issues of further treatment and resuscitation status. Her family members are adamant that she should continue to receive full treatment, be resuscitated in the event of cardiopulmonary arrest and if necessary go to ICU. Her doctors disagree. Who should be making these decisions?
See comment on page 127.

Drugs and treatment

- Several prescribed interventions in resuscitation are not evidence-based.
- Defibrillation, chest compression, assisted ventilation and epinephrine are the present cornerstones of resuscitation.
- Drugs should be administered for specific indications, rather than empirically.
- Safety is essential when using a defibrillator.
- Controversies surrounding resuscitation abound.

Continuity of care

Initiation

The decision about whether to initiate resuscitation is controversial and emotionally fraught. For hospital in-patients a decision should have been reached prior to a cardiac arrest through discussions between the medical staff and the patient and their relatives. Unfortunately, evidence is lacking for doctors' ability to predict outcome from pre-arrest morbidity.

When considering if a 'Do not resuscitate' (DNR) order is appropriate, factors that should be considered include immediate medical problem, medical history and quality of life. Age should not be a determining factor since evidence does not support the commonly held view that the elderly are unlikely to survive an arrest. Many patients do not want to be resuscitated when the probability of survival has been explained to them. Quality of life following resuscitation rather than likelihood of immediate survival may be the most important consideration.

If a DNR order is made it should be clearly documented in the notes, as well as being communicated to all staff members caring for the patient. Where no decision has been taken, resuscitation should proceed until basic facts about the patient are established.

Termination

Having started CPR, a point may be reached when it is considered futile to continue. The whole team should participate in this decision. There is no universally applicable rule; the decision should be taken after persistent failure of treatment of all reversible factors. In most cases resuscitation should be stopped after 30 minutes. However, when cardiac arrest is due to hypothermia or poisoning, patients have survived without neurological impairment after longer attempts.

End tidal carbon dioxide ($ETCO_2$) levels provide an indication of cardiac output during CPR. $ETCO_2$ levels less than 2 KPa (15 mmHg) after 20 minutes of advanced life-support predict death in patients with no pulse but electrical activity on the ECG.

Continuity of care

The return of a palpable cardiac output is not the end-point of resuscitation; it heralds the start of a more challenging phase in the ICU. Good post-resuscitation care is essential, and should start with a detailed history and clinical assessment.

Examination of cardiovascular, respiratory, abdominal and neurological systems may yield clues as to the cause of arrest, for example pitting oedema in congestive cardiac failure or abdominal rigidity if there is intraperitoneal sepsis.

Throughout this period the patient should continue to be closely monitored in terms of cardiac rhythm, haemodynamic status, central venous pressure, blood glucose and arterial blood gases.

Early investigations

- **A**rterial **B**lood gas – Adequacy of ventilation, severity of acidosis and electrolyte derangements.
- **C**hest X-ray – Position of tracheal tube and central venous line. Evidence of trauma, aspiration and cardiac failure (see Fig. 1).
- **D**extrose stix – Treat hypoglycaemia and hyperglycaemia.
- **E**CG – Cardiac rhythm and ischaemia.

Particular attention should be paid to arterial blood gases, especially when mechanical ventilation is employed, since cerebral vasoconstriction may occur if the $PaCO_2$ decreases below 4 KPa (30 mmHg). With such monitoring demands, and as these patients frequently require ventilatory support, further management is best undertaken in the intensive care setting.

Prediction of neurological outcome on the basis of a neurological examination performed immediately after the arrest is impossible. For example, atropine and epinephrine (adrenaline) given during the arrest result in fixed and dilated pupils, which are indistinguishable from a corpse's pupils (see Fig. 2).

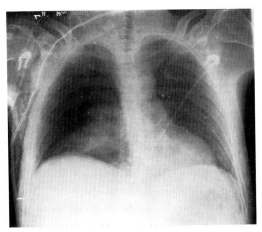

Fig. 1 **CXR showing a large right-sided pneumothorax following successful resuscitation.** Note the correctly positioned tracheal tube, CVP catheter, nasogastric tube and ECG leads, with no evidence of trauma, heart failure or aspiration.

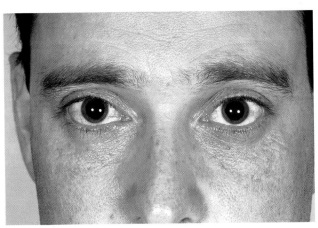

Fig. 2 **Fixed and dilated pupils are not diagnostic of death.**

Airway

Ongoing airway protection is usually necessary. Tracheal tube placement is advisable prior to transfer to the intensive care unit.

Breathing

Assisted ventilation with supplementary oxygen is required. A nasogastric tube should be passed to relieve gastric distension that may have occurred during the initial resuscitation, as air in the stomach may impede effective chest expansion and ventilation.

Circulation

Intravenous access and cardiac monitoring is needed for a minimum of 36 hours.

Rhythm   Patients may require prophylactic anti-arrhythmic therapy to maintain a cardiac rhythm that is compatible with adequate tissue perfusion.

Perfusion pressure   Urine output provides a useful surrogate of adequate vital organ perfusion (and intravascular volume). Hourly urine output should exceed 0.5 ml/kg/hr. Urine output is less useful when there is renal failure.

Central venous pressure   Following a cardiac arrest, cardiac performance is frequently compromised and a CVP catheter (or even a pulmonary artery catheter) may be useful to guide fluid therapy and to infuse inotropes, such as epinephrine (adrenaline).

Thrombolysis   If there is evidence that a myocardial infarction has occurred, thrombolytic therapy is indicated. However, prolonged traumatic CPR is a relative contraindication.

Counselling

Aside from the direct management of the patient post-resuscitation, one of the most important but frequently overlooked aspects of post-resuscitation care is assisting both the patient and the relatives to understand what has happened and the reasons for the actions taken. For those patients who make a full recovery from the event, support may be gained from professional counsellors and a number of self-help groups that have been established.

Breaking bad news

Inevitably not all resuscitations will be successful. A member of the team must take responsibility for telling friends and family that their loved one has died. How, when and where this is done is critical, since it may affect the ability of these people to come to terms with their loss and is likely to be one of the enduring memories of the whole occasion. Below are some suggested tips on how to go about this difficult task, although every health worker may develop their own approach based on personal experience and advice from senior colleagues.

- Take time to consider what has happened and exactly what is to be said to the relatives.
- Find a quiet room where discussions with the relatives can be held.
- It may be helpful if both the doctors and nurses who cared for the patient are present when the news is broken.
- Be prepared to spend time with the relatives and ask a colleague to hold your pager so that you are not disturbed.
- Direct and honest communication leaves no doubt about what has occurred. Euphemisms such as 'passed away' and 'gone to a better place' are best avoided.
- Encourage the relatives to ask questions and admit freely that not all the answers are known.
- Do not be afraid of silent pauses while relatives take in what has been said and be prepared for a full spectrum of emotional responses.
- Explain that relatives are welcome to contact the hospital or the Relative Liaison Officer to answer any further questions.

Clinical Tips on breaking bad news

[Dr Lydgate] said to himself that he was only doing right in telling her the truth about her husband's probable future. A medical man likes to make psychological observations, and sometimes in the pursuit of such studies is too easily tempted into momentous prophesy which life and death easily set at naught. Lydgate had often been satirical on this gratuitous prediction and he meant now to be guarded.

Many of us looking back through life would say that the kindest man we have ever known has been a medical man, or perhaps that surgeon whose fine tact, directed by deeply-informed perception, has come to us in our need with a more sublime beneficence than that of miracle-workers.

From George Eliot's *Middlemarch*, Köneman, Köln, 1997

Continuity of care

- When resuscitation is inappropriate, the 'do not resuscitate' decision should be discussed with all concerned and clearly documented in the patient's notes.
- Resuscitation should be terminated when it is clear that prognosis is poor.
- The standard of care following initial successful resuscitation will determine eventual outcome.
- Counselling and breaking bad news is an essential task for which all members of the team should receive support and training.

Clinical case comments

Clinical case 1
This patient requires reassurance. Surgery and anaesthesia are much safer than in the past. As the operation is minor it is quite possible that use of a laryngoscope will not be necessary, which is often the cause of broken teeth. As regards the penicillin allergy, he will be wearing a bracelet alerting everyone to his allergy and his notes and drug chart will be clearly marked.

Clinical case 2
The patient should be questioned about symptoms. If he is symptom-free, he should be reassured and offered an antacid, like oral ranitidine, prior to surgery. He may take clear oral fluids until 2 hours before the operation. If he is symptomatic expert advice should be sought.

Clinical case 3
She is at risk for DVT and she needs ongoing control of epilepsy.
For DVT prevention:
Stop oral contraceptive for several weeks. Use thrombosis prophylaxis, like low-molecular-weight heparin, perioperatively. Non-pharmacologic prevention, including elastic stockings and early mobilization, is indicated.

- *For epilepsy*: continue *carbamazepine* and check levels preoperatively. Prescribe benzodiazepine as part of premedication.
- *Other considerations*: *carbamazepine* is a liver enzyme inducer. It may increase her anaesthetic and analgesic requirements. There is also increased metabolism of the contraceptive pill. A pregnancy test may be wise.

Clinical case 4
Mr S can only walk 100 metres before being stopped by pain in his legs. The usual symptomatic presentation of coronary artery disease may be obscured by limited exercise capacity due to claudication, and the stress of surgery may be significantly greater than that encountered in daily living. Mr S requires further cardiovascular evaluation.

Clinical case 5
The most likely cause of the fitting is hypoglycaemia. 50 ml of 50% dextrose should be given immediately via the intravenous route. Blood sugar should be measured along with an arterial blood gas. Other emergency resuscitative measures may follow, including the provision of oxygen and assisting with breathing. This is not easy while fitting continues. Diabetic ketoacidosis and hyperosmolar non-ketotic coma must be excluded. If the problem does not resolve and the blood sugar is normal, other diagnoses, like stroke, may be considered. Ongoing seizures are treated as status epilepticus.

Clinical case 6
There is a recent history of recurrent deep venous thromboses with resultant pulmonary emboli. Ongoing warfarin therapy constitutes an unacceptably high risk for bleeding during major surgery. Warfarin should be stopped, but this will leave the patient vulnerable to further thromboses. Several measures should be taken to reduce this risk.

- *Preoperatively*: warfarin should be stopped about 4 days prior to the operation as warfarin has a half-life of about 48–72 hours. Subcutaneous heparin or low-molecular-weight heparin (LMWH) may be administered as an alternative anticoagulant. This may be discontinued at the time of surgery to allow adequate clotting during the operation.
- *Postoperatively*: conservative measures such as the use of TED stockings, good hydration, early mobilization and calf compression devices all help reduce the risk of postoperative venous thrombosis. Intravenous heparinization by infusion should be commenced in the postoperative period until oral anticoagulation has been re-established and the INR reflects an adequate warfarin effect.

Clinical case 7
This woman has a body mass index of 58 kg/m². The waist to hip ratio is 0.92. She is morbidly obese with an unfavourable waist to hip fat distribution. Her risk of having undiagnosed co-existing diseases and of succumbing to perioperative complications is significantly increased. Blood pressure should be rechecked using a large cuff and investigations for co-morbidity are warranted.

Clinical case 8
Physical examination is unreliable in determining satisfactory control in asthma. The operation is elective. Two weeks of oral steroid therapy are indicated after which the peak flow testing and examination may be repeated. If the surgery had been urgent, regional anaesthesia may have been considered.

Clinical case 9
He should immediately wash the area with soap and water and refer to the local hospital policy. Needle-stick injuries are usually reported to the occupational health department, who will then advise on the requirement for further action, such as the administration of triple antiretroviral therapy. Antiretroviral therapy is most effective if commenced within a few hours, so accidents occurring at night should be handled with the same urgency as those occurring during the day. A serum sample should be taken from the donor and recipient. Antibodies for HBV and HCV can be measured. HIV antibody testing usually requires informed consent. Antiretrovirals may be commenced before results of HIV tests are available.

Clinical case 10
Acute alcohol withdrawal is a life-threatening medical emergency. Hypoglycaemia should be excluded. If he is cooperative, treatment could include:

- iv dextrose
- iv thiamine 100 mg plus multivitamins.
- Oral or iv benzodiazepine (lorazepam 1–2 mg).

In patients who are uncooperative, unconscious or fitting, the following is suggested:

- iv access should be obtained
- Give iv 50% dextrose and thiamine.
- Administer 2 mg iv lorazepam.
- If seizures persist administer 1 g iv phenytoin (with cardiac monitoring).
- Provide oxygen and ensure airway is protected.
- Exclude other underlying problems:
  - head injury
  - hypoxia
  - electrolyte derangement

– sepsis
– liver failure, renal failure, metabolic cause
– other drugs or toxins.
■ Transfer to HDU or ICU.

Clinical case 11

Confusion, pecechiae and hypoxia following a long bone fracture are highly suggestive of a fat embolism syndrome. Multiple pulmonary fat emboli result in dead space ventilation and |right heart strain. Acute respiratory distress syndrome is common. Although saturation has improved with supplementary oxygen, there is significantly impaired transfer of oxygen to the blood. This woman needs urgent fixation of her fracture and management on the intensive care unit.

Clinical case 12

There is alkalaemia as the blood pH is > 7.44. The positive base excess suggests a primary metabolic alkalosis and increased PCO_2 is in keeping with compensatory respiratory acidosis. Na^+, K^+ and Cl^- are all slightly decreased and HCO_3^- is increased.

These findings may be explained on the basis of chronic frusemide therapy. There is a loss of Na^+, Cl^-, K^+ and H^+ in the urine. There is also a likely fluid deficit. Appropriate treatment includes slow infusion of potassium chloride and rehydration with normal saline. A potassium-sparing diuretic should be added, or used in place of frusemide.

Clinical case 13

Naloxone will reverse the morphine analgesia and precipitate acute pain, possibly worsening his breathing further. Even without supplementary oxygen, PaO_2 is not very low. There are no apparent untoward effects of the respiratory acidosis. This patient should receive supplementary oxygen. A pulse oximeter may be used to warn of hypoxaemia. Regular monitoring of consciousness level and ventilatory rate is advisable.

Clinical case 14

The most likely cause of her confusion and seizure is hyponatraemia (with cerebral oedema) and fluid overload. Other common causes like hypoxia, hypoglycaemia, acid–base abnormalities, infection, stroke and myocardial infarction should be excluded.

The following steps should be taken:
■ Admit her to a high dependency unit and check plasma sodium concentration.
■ Administer oxygen and institute regular neurological observation.
■ Intravenous hypertonic saline (such as 3% saline) may be given at a rate of no more than 0.5 ml/kg/hr.
■ Sodium correction exceeding 8 mmol/l may result in central pontine myelinolysis.
■ Furosemide may be given if over-hydration is present.

Recheck the sodium at regular intervals and correct other likely electrolyte abnormalities, like hypokalaemia and hypomagnesaemia.

Clinical case 15

Shivering is part of a thermoregulatory reflex to increase core temperature. It can be triggered by a decrease in core temperature such as occurs during surgery or by a re-setting of the 'set-point' in the hypothalamus, such as in an infective fever. In this patient it is important to distinguish between the two because the management is totally different. Measurement of core temperature will reveal the cause of shivering. Hypothermia is more likely in this setting and is treated by applying warming devices to the surface of the body and warming all intravenous and bladder irrigation fluids. Shivering can be attenuated by opioid analgesics. Hypothermia lowers the threshold of pain. If the core temperature is 37°C or higher, sepsis must be considered and treated with appropriate antibiotics. Fever may be treated with paracetamol.

Clinical case 16

Postoperative cognitive dysfunction (POCD) is common in the elderly, but is a diagnosis of exclusion. There may be alarming and even life-threatening reasons underlying agitation and confusion. It is imperative to consider such causes as hypoxia, hypercarbia, hypotension, hypoglycaemia, acid–base disturbance, electrolyte abnormality, alcohol withdrawal, stroke, myocardial infarction, arrhythmia, drug overdose and hypothermia. After excluding a life-threatening emergency, the house officer should seek advice from a senior colleague.

Clinical case 17

Clinical practice would require the parents' presence and the providing of simple explanations. A suitable pre-med could be EMLA® cream and an anxiolytic. Postoperatively, if analgesia has not been prescribed, you would:
■ Clarify analgesia already given in theatre: drug type, dosage, route, time of administration and effect.
■ Obtain the child's weight. Are any drug allergies, any medical contraindications, e.g. asthma and NSAIDs?

Clinical case 18

This women presents with a high risk of bleeding following delivery and of having another blood clot if she stops taking anticoagulant medication. The haematologist should be contacted for a diagnosis and advice, and a consultant obstetrician and anaesthetist should be informed. The INR should be determined, and if it is greater than 1.5, consider intravenous vitamin K 2.5–5 mg iv. Prothrombin factor concentrate (50 units/kg) or fresh frozen plasma (15 ml/kg) may be administered if there is post partum haemorrhage. As soon as bleeding has ceased following delivery, administer heparin or LMWH and re-institute warfarin therapy.

Clinical case 19

The main problems are: obesity, irritable airway due to smoking, procedure usually carried out in the sitting position, possible toxic side-effects of the local anaesthetic instilled into the airway and absent or attenuated airway-protective reflexes following the procedure.

Sedation is best achieved by a trained anaesthetist with an infusion of propofol. The addition of remifentanil to the infusion is advantageous to suppress the cough reflex.

Clinical case 20

Once it is established that the patient is stable and there is no life-threatening problem, patient comfort should be addressed. Adequate analgesia is essential. The pain team may be called to institute epidural analgesia or patient-controlled analgesia. Epidural analgesia not only provides excellent pain relief, but also decreases opiate requirements and may promote bowel motility. An anti-emetic may be prescribed. Active heating is important and a convection warmer could be used to achieve this. Hyperglycaemia requires treatment and enteral feeding with a jejunal tube is warranted as soon as the surgeons feel that this is practical. Other considerations include the prolonged provision of supplementary oxygen, thrombosis prophylaxis and neostigmine to promote bowel decompression.

Clinical case 21

A reasonable approach to endocarditis prophylaxis should take into account the degree to which the underlying condition creates a risk of endocarditis, the risk of bacteraemia associated with the procedure, the potential adverse reactions to the prophylactic agent(s) and cost–benefit aspects.

Rheumatic heart disease is considered a moderate risk for the development of infective endocarditis. High-risk situations include prosthetic heart valves, previous episode of infective endocarditis and complex cyanotic congenital heart disease.

Colonoscopy and upper gastrointestinal endoscopy are associated with bacteraemia in 2–5% of cases and the organisms are unlikely to cause endocarditis. Colonoscopy and biopsy is thus considered a low-risk procedure. In contrast, bacteraemia may occur in 45% of cases of oesophageal dilatation and 31% of cases of sclerotherapy for oesophageal varices.

Antibiotic prophylaxis is not indicated in this instance. However, whenever there is doubt, advice should be sought from a microbiologist or infectious disease physician.

Clinical case 22

Maintenance

- Daily fluid requirements = 1.5 × 80 × 24 = 2880 ml/day. Daily sodium requirements are at least 9 g (more than this may be given, but not less!)
- 1000 ml normal saline 0.9% to run over 8 hours.
- 1000 ml Hartmann's solution to run over 8 hours.
- 1000 ml 5% dextrose to run over 8 hours.

Replacement
Blood loss and fluid sequestration. Crystalloid replacement of blood loss is acceptable, but may require larger volumes. To run concurrently with maintenance fluids:

- 1000 ml of 10% hydroxyethyl starch over 24 hours.

Chart fluid administered and losses (urine and blood) accurately. Re-assess fluid balance at regular intervals (e.g.

8-hourly). Review if blood loss > 500 ml, systolic BP < 90 mmHg, HR > 110 beats/min, CVP < 5 cmH$_2$O or urine output < 40 ml/hour.

Clinical case 23

The transfusion should be temporarily halted and the patient's clinical condition should be assessed. If hypotension is present, the reaction should be treated as anaphylaxis. The unit of blood should be checked again to exclude a mismatch. Acute non-haemolytic transfusion reactions occur commonly (with about 2% of transfusions). Oxygen, paracetamol 1 g, hydrocortisone 100 mg iv and chlorpheniramine 10 mg iv may be administered, and the blood may be trickled in slowly. If there is any suspicion of haemolysis (hypotension, pain, dark urine), stop the blood and send the unit with a blood sample from the patient to the blood bank.

Clinical case 24

Auscultation of both lung fields reveals normal breath sounds on the right side but just audible, wheezy sounds on the left. Pulling out the endotracheal tube by 3 cm restored normal breath sounds on the left side and saturation promptly increased to 99%. A chest X-ray taken immediately after intubation of the trachea shows placement of the tube in the right main bronchus with deviation of the mediastinal shadow to the left.

Clinical case 25

High breathing rate and twitching movements are hallmarks of residual paralysis. Poor oxygenation despite supplementary oxygen and warm peripheries with central hypothermia suggest inadequate ventilation and accumulation of carbon dioxide. Ventilation should be assisted and a blood gas may be informative in revealing the extent of carbon dioxide retention. Help from an anaesthetist is imperative. Clinical weakness revealed by poor hand-grasp and inability to lift the head further suggest the diagnosis. A nerve stimulator also provides valuable information. Residual paralysis may be improved by a cholinesterase inhibitor, such as neostigmine.

Clinical case 26

A patient suffered hypoxaemia (with a peripheral oxygen saturation of 85% on the pulse oximeter) and developed a bradycardia (heart rate decreased to

45 bpm) as a result of a disconnection of the oxygen pipeline supply. This incident resulted from failure to check and maintain the equipment and was exacerbated by inadequate monitoring. The problem was resolved by using an emergency oxygen cylinder.

- Preventability = 1/2 (see comment)
- Outcome = 0
- Critical incident = oxygen supply failure
- Outcome = transient bradycardia and hypoxaemia

Comment
A thorough equipment check might have revealed a loose pipeline connection. An oxygen analyser would have detected the problem more rapidly than a pulse oximeter.

Clinical case 27

The likely diagnosis is an epidural haematoma compressing spinal nerve roots, a surgical emergency. Urgent referral to the neurosurgeons is indicated. Anticoagulation should be reversed with vitamin K to prevent ongoing bleeding. Magnetic resonance imaging may confirm the diagnosis and rapid surgical evacuation of the haematoma could reverse the symptoms.

Clinical case 28

Peripheral vascular disease, coupled with smoking and diabetes, is highly predictive of coronary artery disease. This patient is at risk for myocardial infarction. Hypoxia and hypovolaemia should be rapidly excluded. After it is confirmed that he is breathing, high-concentration oxygen should be administered. A 12-lead ECG, arterial blood gas, haemoglobin and blood samples for cardiac troponin will provide valuable information. Central venous pressure and urine output are useful guides to volume status. After life-threatening causes have been excluded and emergency therapies instituted, senior advice should be sought.

Clinical case 29

Rapid deterioration is possible and two immediate priorities include providing high concentration of oxygen and seeking expert help. Pre-existing cardiopulmonary disease is unlikely. The clinical presentation is consistent with negative pressure pulmonary oedema, which occurs following sustained negative inspiratory pressure against a partially obstructed upper airway, typical of larygospasm. A chest X-ray, central venous line and arterial blood gas may help with the diagnosis and management. This complication is best treated with a period of continuous positive airway pressure (CPAP) or positive pressure ventilation on a high-dependency or intensive care unit.

Clinical case 30

The presentation is highly suggestive of hypovolaemia secondary to blood loss. Immediate priorities include the administration of high-concentration oxygen and 1000 ml of a resuscitation fluid, such as Hartman's solution. Active bleeding should be excluded and haemoglobin concentration determined. If, following these measures, she is still suffering from nausea and is not in pain, cyclizine 50 mg or ondansetron 4 mg iv would be appropriate therapeutic options as she has already received an antidopiminergic medication.

Clinical case 31

Send blood for urgent FBC and clotting tests (INR/APTT) and ensure that at least two units of cross-matched blood are available. Exclude and treat hypothermia and hypertension. Check for residual heparin effect (ACT and APTT or TEG® or HMS®), although this is unlikely 6 hours after surgery. Near-patient assessment of platelet function (PFA-100® or TEG® or HemoSTATUS®) and fibrinolysis (TEG®) may reveal a problem. Antifibrinolytic medications and DDAVP, either guided by haemostatic assessment or administered empirically, may decrease bleeding. Pooled platelets are indicated if the platelet count is < 50 × 10⁹/L or if platelet dysfunction is suspected.Fresh frozen plasma may be administered if laboratory (or near-patient) tests reveal a coagulopathy for which no reversible cause is found. Cryoprecipitate should be given if hypofibrinogenaemia is discovered. Early surgical exploration may identify a specific bleeding point and prevent escalation of the problem.

Clinical case 32

The combination of systemic upset, rigors and fever after intravenous infusion through a central line should raise the suspicion of a line infection. The infusion should be stopped and several sets of blood cultures taken, from peripheral and central sites. Staphylococcal species are the most common causes of infections associated with intravenous lines, but other organisms such as Gram-negative coliforms have been implicated. A suitable empirical regime would be intravenous vancomycin and gentamicin, through a newly sited intravenous line. The tunneled central line should be removed and sent for culture as soon as possible. Following identification of the infecting organism, targeted therapy should be instituted, such as oral ciprofloxacin for coliform infection.

Clinical case 33

Unless it is specified that an item contains no latex, there should be a high index of suspicion. The photograph shows some articles that do contain latex, such as the black rubber and the pale glove. The dark glove and the laryngeal mask do not contain latex. Each hospital should have policy for the management of patients with a suspected latex allergy including a list of latex-free products.

Clinical case 34

Single CVP readings do not provide as much information as trends in CVP values. It is important to confirm that the tip of the CVP catheter is appropriately positioned and that the lumen is patent. The CVP measurements should be made with the patient lying flat and the base of the column or the transducer bridge placed at the level of the heart. A fluid challenge is indicated in this circumstance. Following 250 ml of intravenous fluid (such as normal saline or hydroxyethyl starch), if there is no increase in the central venous pressure, hypovolaemia is likely. A sustained increase of 2–3 cmH$_2$O mitigates against hypovolaemia. A relatively high CVP reading despite hypovolaemia may occur in several situations, such as chronic lung disease with right heart failure.

Clinical case 35

Part 1 Postoperative pain assessment. Ensure PCA is correctly prescribed and attached. Quantify how much analgesia the patient has received so far. Exclude surgical causes (examine the patient/is the patient bleeding?). Once satisfied no acute remediable cause, titrate to comfort. (e.g. 1–2 mg intravenous morphine every few minutes). Add in adjuvant analgesia such as NSAIDs/paracetamol (e.g. diclofenac sodium 50 mg po/pr 8-hourly). Prescribe an anti-emetic (e.g. ondansetron 4 mg iv 8-hourly as required). Re-assess new treatment effect. Contact Acute Pain Team for advice if available.

Part 2 Either opioid overdose or other cause (? hypovolaemic shock). How much opioid has the patient had? Is the patient in clinical shock? Does the patient have a medical condition which would make them more susceptible to opioids? Look for signs of obvious bleeding. Is the patient tachycardic, hypotensive, dilated pupils, reduced/absent urine output, e.g. renal impairment. Are there signs of opioid overdose? Is the patient diabetic? What is the blood glucose? Pin-point pupils, slow respiratory rate (< 8/minute). If opioid overdose suspected discontinue the PCA.

Airway: is the patient maintaining her own airway and is it clear? Support if necessary. Breathing: is the patient making adequate respiratory effect? Administer 100% oxygen and assist breathing if required. Give 400 μg naloxone intravenously. Observe effort. Give further dose of naloxone if required.

(Clinical note: the effect of naloxone may wear off before plasma levels of the opioid fall to an non-dangerous level. BEWARE: signs of opioid overdose may redevelop. The patient must be closely monitored and further doses of naloxone given (either as a bolus or by infusion) as required.)

Circulation: treat hypovolaemia if present. Give 2 litres crystalloid rapidly then reassess. Naloxone will reverse the analgesic effect of the opioid and the patient may then experience pain, with tachycardia and hypertension. Consider treating with a NSAID while naloxone is still present in the system. Re-evaluate treatment.

Clinical case 36

1) Pump placed above chest height.
2) Hand-set out of patients reach.
3) One-way valve incorrectly set up. 4) iv insertion site covered up/infected/kinked. 5) Patient in obvious distress.

Clinical case 37

Likely diagnosis is complex regional pain syndrome, type I. This commonly occurs post wrist fracture, especially in women. Current analgesia is not effective. Think analgesic ladder. She could increase her co-codamol to take 8 tablets per day, however CRPS is a neuropathic pain condition and frequently unresponsive to opioid analgesia. Referral to a chronic pain specialist is advisable. Adjuvant analgesics should be incorporated into her treatment, e.g. amitriptyline 25–100 mg or gabapentin 1–2 g.

Regional analgesic block of the brachial plexus would enable passive physiotherapy to be performed. Increasing mobility and function can dramatically improve CRPS. Reduction of the sympathetic component will be important if the pain is sympathetically maintained. This can be done by performing an intravenous guanethidine block or a stellate ganglion block. An intravenous guanethidine block is performing in a manner identical to that of a Bier's block but 20 mg of guanethidine is added to the prilocaine local anaesthetic (see 'Regional anaesthesia' on pages 90–91 for method).

Clinical case 38

Factors: ischaemic leg pain, angina. Emotional component: fear about losing limb, altered body image, separation from friends (short-term) by hospitalization and (long-term) by isolation. Best option: epidural. Reasons: regional technique with less effect on respiratory system than opioids. Continuous technique providing constant analgesia pre-, intra- and postoperatively. Pre-emptive analgesia: short-term less pain, reduced chest infections and reduced DVT, possibly long-term reduced stump and phantom limb pain. Risk-factors: age, smoking, widespread vascular disease. Stump pain, phantom limb pain, depression, smoking-related (further amputation, lung cancer, CVA, MI). (Refer to pages 65, 81 and 93.)

Clinical case 39

The patient's primary concerns are going to be the inability to move his legs. This is no doubt distressing, however not necessarily unexpected. Although it is the analgesic component of a regional technique that is most often sought, in practice, this is almost impossible to achieve in isolation, as peripheral nerves are made up of motor, sensory and autonomic nerve fibres. Analgesia does, however, tend to be one of the first manifestations of a successful nerve block, rather than say, the absence of motor function. This is due to differential sensitivity of nerve fibres.

Clinically, small unmyelinated B and C fibres appear most sensitive to local anaesthetic blockade. In contrast the large myelinated A fibres require that

much larger a surface area and length be blocked, before conduction is interrupted. In practice this means that the small temperature and pinprick-sensitive pain fibres are anaesthetized before the proprioceptive and motor fibres. The change in motor function can be attributed to the continuous infusion of bupivacaine. This should be explained and the patient should be reassured that he will regain normal movement once the epidural infusion is stopped. However, a sudden change in motor ability could be suggestive of something more sinister, if unrelated to additional local anaesthetic being administered. Remember a technique-related complication is possible, such as direct trauma to the spinal cord or a haematoma. If suspected, contact the anaesthetist who performed the block (or the on-call anaesthetist if out-of-hours) for an urgent review. An urgent MRI may need to be performed as early surgical intervention is necessary to prevent permanent damage.

A full neurological examination of the lower limbs and abdomen is indicated. This includes power and sensation, pinprick (superficial pain), proprioception and deep pain. This should be performed twice and a comparison made to detect further deterioration or improvement of motor function. The level of the block can be established by dermatomal innervation as shown in Fig. 1 on page 103.

The patient's BP has also dropped substantially. This may be due to the epidural blockade causing vasodilatation. This can be combated by raising the patient's legs and increasing the rate of his intravenous fluid infusion. Oxygen should be given to prevent hypoxia and his BP continue to be monitored closely. If his BP fails to respond to fluid administration or there is a further fall in BP, stop epidural infusion and consider administering a vasoconstrictor agent, e.g. ephedrine 3 mg iv bolus (titrate to effect). Seek senior advice as the patient could also be bleeding (only a few hours postop). Treatment must address this possible complication.

Clinical case 40

Consider the role of NSAIDs in precipitating renal failure and stop giving these in the setting of oliguria and increased creatinine at Day 1. Recognize at day 3 that the ileus is failing to resolve and that respiratory function is compromised by increased abdominal

pressure and/or fluid overload in the face of ongoing intravenous fluid administration in a patient with oliguria. Consider at this point the need for central venous pressure monitoring. Measure chloride in case this is contributing to the acidosis. At day 3 recognize that he is very ill and oxygenation and pH are probably within the normal range only by virtue of hyperventilation. He urgently requires ICU/HDU care at this point.

Clinical case 41

There are a number of important lessons. Monitors such as the pulse oximeter are not always reliable and clinical judgement is invaluable. A simple stethoscope may have provided more useful information, for example in diagnosing a pneumothorax, than a pulse oximeter. Institution of invasive monitoring, such as central line insertion, is time-consuming and should not take precedence over acute resuscitation. These procedures have complications, such as pneumothorax and arrhythmia, and should only be attempted by those with the necessary experience. Monitoring by no means guarantees patient safety. Although appropriate monitors were used, intravenous sedation was wholly inappropriate in this patient who was unstable and agitated, probably as a result of hypoxia. Unless there was obvious bleeding, continued resuscitation with volume coupled with increased oxygen therapy would have dramatically improved the patient's condition and allowed time for sober assessment and appropriate management.

Clinical case 42

This man presented with a condition which could render him brain stem-dead. He is now comatose on a ventilator. He has received sedative and neuromuscular blocking drugs, and these must be allowed sufficient time to wear off. He may also be hypothermic, and in need of active warming. This patient should be managed in the intensive care unit until it is clear that his condition is not due to drugs, hypothermia or any other disturbance. Once brain stem death is confirmed the family may be approached about the possibility of organ donation.

Clinical case 43

The priority is oxygenation, not intubation. The SHO should be informed clearly that the patient's life is in imminent jeopardy. Urgent ventilation using a bag and mask with supplementary oxygen is indicated. If ventilation is sub-optimal despite insertion of a Guedel oropharyngeal airway, placement of a laryngeal mask airway may facilitate airflow to the lungs. Repeated intubation attempts cause swelling which may precipitate airway obstruction.

Clinical case 44

The key to successful outcome is early defibrillation. CPR buys time, but the cardiac arrest was witnessed and the defibrillator is to hand. Precordial thump and chest compressions may disrupt or damage bypass grafts. For this patient, defibrillation (three shocks) is the first choice prior to instituting CPR. If immediate defibrillation is successful, oxygen should be provided and a cause of electrical instability, like hypokalaemia, should be sought and treated. Specific circumstances inform management during a cardiac arrest.

Clinical case 45

There are no easy answers to such ethical dilemmas. Poor communication may underpin the different outlooks of the family members and the physicians. There may be value in holding discussions together with a third party, such as a social worker or a counsellor. Consensus should be sought. The woman described has a very poor prognosis and invasive therapy, such as mechanical ventilation, seems inappropriate. Most families will not wish their loved ones to experience pointless prolonged suffering and would prefer them to die with dignity. Following frank and honest discussion, it is likely that agreement on palliative care will be reached.

Further reading

Perioperative medications
Drugs and Therapeutics Bulletin 1999; 37(8): 62–64

Perioperative safety
http://www.gmc-uk.org
http://www.the-mdu.com

Diabetes mellitus

Bolli GB, Fanelli CG. Unawareness of hypoglycemia. New England Journal of Medicine 1995; 333(26): 1771

Clark CM Jr, Lee DA. Drug therapy: prevention and treatment of the complications of diabetes mellitus. New England Journal of Medicine 1995; 332(18): 1210

Mandrup-Poulsen T. Diabetes recent advances. British Medical Journal 1998; 316: 1221–1225

Obesity
Hunter J, Reid C. Anaesthetic management of the morbidly obese patient. Hospital Medicine 1998; 59(6): 481–483

Stunkard AJ. Current views on obesity. American Journal of Medicine 1996; 100: 230–235 (http://www.gasnet.org)

Pulmonary disease
Smetana GW. Preoperative pulmonary evaluation. New England Journal of Medicine 1999; 340(12): 937–944

HIV and other viruses
Avidan MS, Jones N, Pozniak AL. The implications of HIV for the anaesthetist and intensivist. Anaesthesia 2000; 55: 344–354

Department of Health. Guidelines on Post Exposure Prophylaxis for Health Care Workers Occupationally exposed to HIV. London: Department of Health, 1997

Perspectives in Disease Prevention and Health Promotion. Universal precautions for prevention of transmission of HIV, Hepatitis B and other blood-borne pathogens in a health care setting. Morbidity and Mortality Weekly Reports 1988; 37(24): 377–388

Zuckerman AJ, Harrison TJ, Zuckerman JN. Viral hepatitis. In: Cook GC (ed) Manson's Tropical Diseases 20th edn. London: WB Saunders, 1996: pp 666–685

Alcohol and substance misuse
Tonnesen H, Kehlet H. Preoperative alcoholism and postoperative morbidity. British Journal of Surgery 1999; 86: 869–874

Tonnesen H, Rosenberg J. Effect of preoperative abstinence on poor postoperative outcome in alcohol misusers: randomised controlled trial. British Medical Journal 1999; 318: 1311–1316

Wood PR, Soni N. Anaesthesia and substance abuse. Anaesthesia 1989; 44: 869–874

Oxygen and hypoxia
Lavery GG. Fear of hypercapnia is leading to inadequate oxygen treatment. British Medical Journal 1999; 318: 872

Leach RM, Treacher DF. ABC of oxygen. Oxygen transport 2. Tissue hypoxia. British Medical Journal 1998; 317(14): 1370–1373

Treacher DF, Leach RM. ABC of oxygen: Oxygen transport 1. Basic principles. British Medical Journal 1998; 317(7): 1302–1306

Acid–base abnormalities
Adrogue HJ, Madias NE. Management of life-threatening acid–base disorders. New England Journal of Medicine 1998; 338: 26–34

Kellum JA. Determinants of blood pH in health and disease. Critical Care 2000; 4: 6–14

http://www.anaesthetist.com (excellent overviews of acid–base)

Carbon dioxide
Gluck SL. Electrolyte quintet: Acid–base. Lancet 1998; 352: 474–479

Laffey JG, Kavanagh BP. Carbon dioxide and the critically ill – too little of a good thing? Lancet 1999; 354: 1283–1286

West JB. Respiratory Physiology – the Essentials. 5th edn. Baltimore: Williams & Wilkins, 1995

Electrolytes
Androgue HJ, Madias NE. Primary Care: Hypernatremia. New England Journal of Medicine 2000; 342: 1493–1500

Androgue HJ, Madias NE. Primary Care: Hyponatremia. New England Journal of Medicine 2000; 342: 1581–1589

Bushinsky DA, Monk RD. Electrolyte quintet: Calcium. Lancet 1998; 352: 305–311

Halperin ML, Kamel KS. Electrolyte quintet: Potassium. Lancet 1998; 352: 135–140

Kumar S, Berl T. Electrolyte quintet: Sodium. Lancet 1998; 352

Weisinger JR, Bellorín-Font E. Electrolyte quintet: Magnesium and phosphorus. Lancet 1998; 352: 391–396

Temperature
Sessler DI. Perioperative heat balance. Anesthesiology 2000; 92: 578–596

Sessler DI. Mild perioperative hypothermia. New England Journal of Medicine 1997; 336: 1730–1737

The elderly
Bedford PD. Adverse cerebral effects of anaesthesia on old people. Lancet 1955; 2: 257–263

Infants and children
Cohen MM, Cameron CB. Should you cancel the operation if the child has an upper respiratory tract infection? Anesthesia and Analgesia 1991; 72: 282–288

Cote CJ. Pre-operative preparation and premedication. British Journal of Anaesthesia 1999; 83(1): 16–28

Pregnancy and childbirth
von Dadelszen P, Ornstein MP, Bull SB, Logan AG, Koren G, Magee LA. Fall in mean arterial pressure and fetal growth restriction in pregnancy hypertension: a meta-analysis. Lancet 2000; 355: 87–92

Greer IA. Thrombosis series: Thrombosis in pregnancy: maternal and fetal issues. Lancet 1999; 353: 1258–1265

Halpern SH, Leighton BL, Ohlsson A, Barrett JFR, Rice A. Effect of epidural vs parenteral opioid analgesia on the progress of labor a meta-analysis. Journal of the American Medical Association 1998; 280: 2105–2110

Sibai BH. Drug therapy: treatment of hypertension in pregnant women. New England Journal of Medicine 1996; 335(4)

Sedation
Ponte J, Craig DC. Sedation. Dental Update 1988; 31(Sppt III): 6

The stress response
Kehlet H. Multimodal approach to control postoperative pathophysiology and rehabilitation. British Journal of Anaesthesia 1997; 78: 606–617

Mayers I, Johnson D. The nonspecific inflammatory response to injury. Canadian Journal of Anaesthesia 1998; 45(9): 871–879

Antibiotic prophylaxis
Dajani AS, Taubert KA, Wilson W et al. Prevention of bacterial endocarditis. Recommendations of the American Heart Society. Journal of the American Medical Association 1997; 277(22): 1794–1801

Greif R, Akca O, Horn E-P, Kurz A, Sessler DI. Supplemental perioperative oxygen to reduce the incidence of surgical-wound infection. New England Journal of Medicine 2000; 342: 161–7.

Kernodle DS, Kaiser AB Postoperative infections and antimicrobial prophylaxis. In: Mandell GL, Bennett JE, Dolin R (eds) Principles and Practice of Infectious Diseases, 4th edn. New York: Churchill Livingstone, 1995: pp 2742–2756

Melling AC, Ali B, Scott EM, Leaper DJ. Effects of post-operative warming on the incidence of wound infection after clean surgery: a randomized controlled trial. Lancet 2001; 358: 876–80.

International Symposium on Perioperative Antibiotic Prophylaxis. Section 1: Theoretical and preclinical experimental bases of prophylaxis and Section 2: Clinical uses of prophylaxis. Reviews of Infectious Diseases 1991; 13(Spp10): S779– S873

Reese RE, Betts RF. Antibiotic use, prophylactic antibiotics. In: Reese RE, Betts RF (eds) A Practical Approach to Infectious Diseases, 4th edn. New York: Little Brown and Company, 1996: pp 1097–1121

Van der Berghe G, Wouters P, Weekers F, Verwast C, Bruyninckx F, Schetz M, Vlasselaers D, Ferdinande P, Lauwers P, Bouillon R. Intensive insulin therapy in critically ill patients. New England Journal of Medicine. 2001; 345: 1359–67.

Fluid management
Schierhout G, Roberts I. Fluid resuscitation with colloid or crystalloid solutions in critically ill patients: a systematic review of randomised trials. British Medical Journal 1998; 316: 961–964

Blood products
Goodnough LT, Brecher ME, Kanter MH, AuBuchon. Transfusion medicine – blood transfusion. New England Journal of Medicine 1999; 340(6): 438–447

Goodnough LT, Brecher ME, Kanter MH, AuBuchon. Transfusion medicine – blood conservation. New England Journal of Medicine 1999; 340(7): 525–533

Oximetry and capnography
Brodski JB. What intra-operative monitoring makes sense? Chest 1999; 115: 101S–105S

Duncan PG, Cohen MM. Pulse oximetry and capnography in anaesthetic practice: an epidemiological appraisal. Canadian Journal of Anaesthesia 1991; 38: 619–625

Williams AJ. ABC of oxygen: assessing and interpreting arterial blood gases and acid base balance. British Medical Journal 1988; 317: 1213–1216

Postoperative recovery
Association of Anaesthetists of Great Britain and Ireland. Immediate Postanaesthetic Recovery, 1993

Intraoperative complications
www.rcoa.ac.uk/critincident/ciweb.html

Postoperative nausea and vomiting
Baines MJ. ABC of palliative care: Nausea, vomiting, and intestinal obstruction. British Medical Journal 1997; 315: 1148–1150

Langer RA. Postoperative Nausea and Vomiting. http://gasnet.med.yale.edu/gta/nausea.html

Postoperative bleeding
Despotis GJ, Gravlee G, Filos K, Levy J. Anticoagulation monitoring during cardiac surgery: a review of current and emerging techniques. Anesthesiology 1999; 91(4): 1122–1151

Despotis GJ, Levine V, Saleem R, Spitznagel E, Joist JH. Use of point-of-care test in identification of patients who can benefit from desmopressin during cardiac surgery: a randomised controlled trial. Lancet 1999; 354(9173): 106–110

Shore Lesserson L, Manspeizer HE, DePerio M, Francis S, Vela Cantos F, Ergin MA. Thromboelastography-guided transfusion algorithm reduces transfusions in complex cardiac surgery. Anesthesia and Analgesia 1999; 88(2): 312–319

Perioperative infection
Damani NN. (1997). Manual of Infection Control Procedures. Prevention of Infection Associated with Urinary Catheter. London: Greenwich Medical Media Ltd, 1999: pp 170–173

Girgawy E, Raad I (1999). Catheter-related infections. In: Wilcox MH (ed) Fast facts – Infection Highlights 1998–99. Oxford: Health Press Ltd, 1999: pp 73–81

Worsley MA. Infection control and prevention of Clostridium difficile infection. Journal of Antimicrobial Chemotherapy 1998; 41(Sppt C): S59–S66

Young PJ, Ridley SA. Ventilator-associated pneumonia. Anaesthesia 1999; 54: 1183–1197

Allergic reactions
ABC of allergies. Anaphylaxis. British Medical Journal 1998; 316: 1442–1445

Suspected Anaphylactic Reactions Associated with Anaesthesia. Association of Anaesthetist Guidelines, 1995. http://gasnet.med.yale.edu/gta/late

Pain assessment, measurement and documentation
Ashari MA, Nocholas MK. Personality and adjustment to chronic pain. Pain Reviews 1999; 6: 85–97

C de C Williams A. Pain measurement in chronic pain management. Pain Reviews 1995; 2: 39–63

Post JM, Robins RS. When Illness Strikes the Leader. New Haven: Yale University Press, 1993

Royal College of Surgeons of England and the College of Anaesthetists. Report of the Working Party on Pain after Surgery. London: Royal College of Surgery, 1990

Pain definitions and physiology
Serpell M, Mackin A, Harvey A. Acute pain physiology and pharmacological tartgets: The future and present. International Journal of Acute Pain Management 1998; 1(3): 31–47

Woolf CJ, Mannion RT. Neuropathic pain: aetiology, symptoms, mechanisms and management. Lancet 1999; 353(9168): 1959–1964

Pharmacological intervention in pain management

Kam PCA. Cyclo-oxygenase isoenzymes: physiological and pharmacological role. Anaesthesia 2000; 55: 442–449

McQuay H. Opioids in pain management. Lancet 1999; 353(9171): 2229–2232

Acute pain management

Rawal N. Postoperative pain and its management. In: Rawa N (ed) Management of Acute and Chronic Pain. London: BMJ Books, 1998: pp 51–58

Royal College of Surgeons of England and the College of Anaesthetists. Report of the Working Party on Pain after Surgery. London: Royal College of Surgery, 1990

Patient-controlled analgesia

Ferrante FM, Ostheimer GW, Ovino BG. Patient Controlled Analgesia. Oxford: Blackwell Scientific Publications, 1990

Local anaesthesia

Lonsdale M, Buckley JR, Macrae WA. Local anaesthesia for the non-anaesthetist. Hospital Update 1991; 229–236

Regional anaesthesia

Wildsmith JAW, Armitage EN (eds) Principles and Practice of Regional Anaesthesia. Edinburgh, Churchill Livingstone, 1987

Chronic pain syndromes

Andersson GB. Epidemiological features of chronic low-back pain. Lancet 1999; 354(9178): 581–585

Ashburn MA, Staats PS. Management of chronic pain. Lancet 1999; 353(9167): 1865–1869

Sherman RA. What do we really know about phantom limb pain? Pain Reviews 1994; 4: 261–274

Complementary medicine and analgesia

Kumar RN, Chamber WA, Pertwee RG. Pharmacological actions and therapeutic uses of cannabis and cannabinoids. Anaesthesia 2001; 56: 1059–1068.

ZollmanC, Vickers A. ABC of Complementary Medicine. London: BMJ Books, 2000

ABCDs of pain management problems

Avidan MS, Jones N, Poznik AL. The implications of HIV for the anaesthetist and the intensivist. Anaesthesia 2000; 55: 344–354

Pain in the young and the old

Harkins SW. Price DD. Bush FM, et al. Geriatric pain. In: Wall PD, Melzack R (eds) Textbook of Pain. Edinburgh: Churchill Livingstone, 1994

Lloyd-Thomas A. Assessment and control of pain in children. Anaesthesia 1995; 50: 753–755

Morton NS. Prevention and control of pain in children. British Journal of Anaesthesia 1999; 83(1): 118–129

Cancer pain management

Portenoy RK, Lesage P. Management of cancer pain. Lancet 2000; 353(9165): 1695–1700

Useful advice for house officers and non-anaesthetists

Finucane BT (ed) Complications of Regional Anaesthesia. Pennsylvania: Churchill Livingstone, 1999

What is intensive care?

ABC of Intensive Care. BMJ 1999; 318(7196–7207)

Goldhill DR, White SA, Summer A. Physiological values and procedures in the 24 h before ICU admission from the ward, Anaesthesia 1999; 54(6): 529–534.

Goldhill DR, Worthington L, Mulcahy A, Tarling M, Summer A. The patient at-risk team: identifying and managing seiously ill ward patients. Anaesthesia 1999; 54(9): 853–860

Reasons for ICU admission

Adam S, Forrest S. ABC of intensive care: Other supportive care. British Medical Journal 1999; 319: 175–178

Grant IS, Andrews PJD. ABC of intensive care: Neurological support. British Medical Journal 1999; 319: 110–113

Smith G, Nielsen M. ABC of intensive care: Criteria for admission. British Medical Journal 1999; 318: 1544–1547

Brain death and organ donation

Pallis C, Harley DH. ABC of Brainstem Death, 2nd Edn. London: BMJ publishing group

Psychological aspects of ICU

Eddleston JM, White P, Guthrie E. Survival, morbidity and quality of life after discharge from intensive care. Critical Care Medicine 2000; 28(7): 2293–2299

Winter B, Cohen S. ABC of intensive care: Withdrawal of treatment. 1999; 319(7205): 306–308

Abbreviations

ACE	angiotensin converting enzyme
ACT	activated clotting time
ACTH	adrenocorticotrophic hormone
ADH	antidiuretic hormone
AG	anion gap
APTT	activated partial thromboplastin time
ARDS	acute respiratory distress syndrome
ART	antiretroviral therapy
ASA	American Society of Anesthesiologists
AT	arterial thrombosis
BBB	blood brain barrier
BMI	body mass index
BP	blood pressure
BSI	blood stream infection
CAG	coronary artery graft
CDAD	*Clostridium difficile* associated diarrhoea
CI	plasma chloride
CNS	central nervous system
CO	carbon monoxide or cardiac output
COPD	chronic obstructive pulmonary disease
CPAP	continuous positive airway pressure
CPP	cerebral perfusion pressure
CPR	cardiopulmonary resuscitation
CRP	C-reactive protein
CRPS	complex regional pain syndrome
CSF	cerebrospinal fluid
CT	computerised tomography
CTZ	chemoreceptor trigger zone
CVA	cerebrovascular accident
CXR	chest radiograph
DIC	disseminated intravascular coagulation
DKA	diabetic ketoacidosis
DPG	diphosphoglycerate
DVT	deep venous thrombosis
ECG	electrocardiograph
ERCP	endoscopic retrograde cholangiopancreatography
ESR	erythrocyte sedimentation rate
$ETCO_2$	end tidal carbon dioxide
FBC	full blood count

FFP	fresh frozen plasma
FiO_2	fraction of inspired oxygen
FIX	coagulation factor IX
FVIII	coagulation factor VIII
GA	general anaesthesia
HAI	hospital acquired infection
Hb	haemoglobin
HBcAg	HBV core antigen
HBIG	human HBV immunoglobulin
HbO_2	oxyhaemoglobin
Hb-red	deoxyhaemoglobin
HBsAg	HBV surface antigen
HBV	hepatitis B virus
HCO_3	plasma bicarbonate
HCO_{3a}	actual plasma bicarbonate
HCO_{3s}	standard plasma bicarbonate
HCV	hepatitis C virus
HDL	high density lipoprotein
HDU	high dependency unit
HIV	human immunodeficiency virus
HR	heart rate (beats per minute)
IASP	International Association for the Study of Pain
ICP	intracranial pressure
ICU	intensive care unit
IE	infective endocarditis
im	intramuscular administration of drug
INR	international normalised ratio
IPPV	intermittent positive pressure ventilation
iv	intravenous administration of drug
JVP	jugular venous pressure
K	plasma potassium
LA	local anaesthetic
LDL	low density lipoprotein
LMA	laryngeal mask airway
LMWH	low molecular weight heparin
MAOI	monoamine oxide inhibitor
MAP	mean arterial pressure
MI	myocardial infarction
MRI	magnetic resonance imaging
MRSA	methicillin resistant *Staphylococcus aureus*
MSU	mid stream urine
N_2O	nitrous oxide
Na	plasma sodium
NSAID	non steroidal anti-

	inflammatory drug
$PaCO_2$	partial pressure of carbon dioxide (arterial)
PaO_2	partial pressure of oxygen (arterial)
PAP	pulmonary artery pressure
PCA	patient controlled analgesia
PCEA	patient controlled epidural anaesthesia
pCO_2	partial pressure of carbon dioxide
PCR	polymerase chain reaction
PCS	patient controlled sedation
PCWP	pulmonary capillary wedge pressure
PDPH	post dural puncture headache
PE	pulmonary embolism
PEEP	positive end expiratory pressure
PG	prostaglandin
po	oral administration of drug
pO_2	partial pressure of oxygen
POCD	postoperative cognitive dysfunction
PONV	postoperative nausea and vomiting
PTCA	percutaneous transluminal coronary angioplasty
RR	respiratory rate (breaths per minute)
sc	subcutaneous administration of drug
SMP	sympathetically maintained pain
SSI	surgical site infection
SV	stroke volume
TCA	tricyclic antidepressant
TEG	thromboelastograph
TPN	total parenteral nutrition
TRALI	transfusion related acute lung injury
TURP	transurethral resection of prostate
URTI	upper respiratory tract infection
UTI	urinary tract infection
VC	vomiting centre
VF	ventricular fibrillation
VWF	Von Willebrand's factor
WHO	World Health organisation
WHR	waist:hip ratio

Subject Index

Abbreviations used in this index include:-
HDU–High dependency unit
ICU–Intensive care unit
PCA–Patient-controlled analgesia
PONV–Postoperative nausea and vomiting

A

ABC resuscitation 119
acetylcholine, temperature regulation 34
acidaemia
 definition 28
 problems due to 28
 in resuscitation 118
 treatment 28–29
acid–base abnormalities 28–29
 clinical case 29, 123
 diagnosis 29
 drugs associated 29
 postoperative arrhythmias 64
 see also acidosis; alkalosis
acidosis
 definition 28
 metabolic *see* metabolic acidosis
 respiratory 28
acupressure 68, 69
acupuncture 94
 mechanism of action 94
acute pain *see* pain
acute pain team 85
acute renal failure (ARF), common causes 107
acute respiratory distress syndrome (ARDS)
 management 106
 postoperative 66, 67
 shock 77
 underlying pathology 67
acyclovir, analgesia in AIDS patients 96
adenosine, resuscitation 118
adjuvant analgesics 83
 burns patients 97
adrenaline (epinephrine)
 allergy treatment 75
 local infiltration 90
 nerve blocks 91
 resuscitation 118
α-2 adrenergic agonists
 analgesic effects 83
 myocardial ischaemia prevention 65
β-adrenergic blockers *see* beta-blockers
aerobic respiration, mitochondria 27
affective pain, definition 80
AIDS patients
 analgesia 96
 pain symptoms 96
 treatment goals 96
 see also HIV
airway management
 emergency 114–115
 post-resuscitation 121
airway obstruction, postoperative 66
airways integrity/patency, recovery room function 56
alcohol
 acute intoxication 24
 metabolism 24
 teratogenicity 40
 units 24
 withdrawal 24
alcohol abuse 24–25
 anaesthetic resistance 24
 analgesic resistance 24
 clinical case 25, 122–123
 postoperative morbidity 25
 surgical morbidity 24
alkalaemia
 definition 28
 problems 29
alkali therapy, acidaemia 28
alkalosis
 definition 28
 metabolic *see* metabolic alkalosis
 respiratory 29, 31
allergen, definition 74
allergic reactions 74–75
 clinical case 75, 125
 definition and key terms 74
 diagnosis 75
 pathology 74
 prevention 75
 risk in hospitalized patients 74–75
 treatment 75
allergies, preoperative assessment 6
allodynia 80, 81
alpha-2 adrenergic agonists
 analgesic effects 83
 myocardial ischaemia prevention 65
alveolar ventilation 30
American Society of Anesthesiologists (ASA)
 preoperative physical status classification 7
 sedation recommendations 44–45
amethocaine 39, 88
amitriptyline, postoperative neuralgia 92
amputation, phantom limb pain 93
anaemic hypoxia 26–27
anaesthesia
 alcohol resistance 24
 balanced 42
 elderly patients 37
 infants/children 39
 mortality associated 4
 recovery 42
 see also general anaesthesia; regional anaesthesia
anaesthetic techniques 42–43
 decision-making 43
 elderly patients 37
 history of perioperative care 2–3
 options 42
anaesthetists
 childbirth 41
 role in surgery 5
analgesia
 administration in infants/children 98
 elderly patients 37
 methods 84–85
 patient controlled *see* patient controlled analgesia (PCA)
 Rule of Fives 83
analgesics
 adjuvant 83
 administration routes 85
 alcohol resistance 24
 drug-related problems 102
 ideal properties 84
 important targets 81
 non-opioid analgesics 82
 opioid analgesics *see* opioid analgesics
 technique-related problems 102
 WHO prescribing ladder 100
 see also individual drugs
anaphylactoid reaction 74
 features 75
anaphylaxis 74
 features 75
angiotensin converting enzyme (ACE) inhibitors
 perioperative use 8
 teratogenicity 40
anion gap (AG) 28
antibiotic(s)
 history of perioperative care 3
 spectrum 48–49
antibiotic prophylaxis
 cephalosporins 48–49
 clinical case 49, 124
 duration 49
 regimens 49
 surgical site infection 48–49
 timing 49
antibody, definition 74
anticholinergic drugs
 PONV treatment 69
 postoperative cognitive dysfunction 37
anticoagulants, perioperative use 9
anticoagulation
 perioperative management 17
 reversal 16
anticonvulsants
 analgesic effects 83
 postoperative neuralgia 92
antidepressants
 analgesic effects 83
 perioperative use 9
 see also tricyclic antidepressants (TCAs)
antidiuretic hormone, surgical stress response 50
antidopaminergic drugs, PONV treatment 69
antiemetics
 metabolic alkalosis treatment 29
 patient-controlled analgesia and 87
 PONV treatment 69
anti-epileptic drugs, teratogenicity 40
antihistaminergic drugs, PONV treatment 69
antipyretics 35
antiretroviral therapy (ART), HIV 22
antisepsis, history of perioperative care 3
antispasmodics, opiate withdrawal 97
α-1 antitrypsin deficiency 21
aortic regurgitation, surgical complications 10
aortic stenosis, severe, surgical complications 10
arrhythmias
 control 10
 management algorithm 65
 postoperative 64
 predisposing factors 64
arterial blood gases
 analysis 28
 ICU patient monitoring 108
 investigation after resuscitation 120
 lung function assessment 20
arterial blood pressure *see* blood pressure
arterial blood sampling, practical procedure 59
arterial thromboses 16
aspiration, gastric contents *see* gastric contents aspiration
aspirin
 perioperative use 8
 temperature regulation 35